Thou Shalt Never Get Rid of Us

Thou Shalt Never Get Rid of Us

25 years quarreling with voices

MIGUEL ASECAS

Copyright © 2021 Miguel Asecas
Originally published in Spain under the title: *Nunca te librarás de nosotros* (Caligrama 2020)
Covert Art: Carlos Pueyo and Miguel Asecas

The moral right of the author has been asserted.

Apart from any fair dealing for the purposes of research or private study, or criticism or review, as permitted under the Copyright, Designs and Patents Act 1988, this publication may only be reproduced, stored or transmitted, in any form or by any means, with the prior permission in writing of the publishers, or in the case of reprographic reproduction in accordance with the terms of licences issued by the Copyright Licensing Agency. Enquiries concerning reproduction outside those terms should be sent to the publishers.

Matador
9 Priory Business Park,
Wistow Road, Kibworth Beauchamp,
Leicestershire. LE8 0RX
Tel: 0116 279 2299
Email: books@troubador.co.uk
Web: www.troubador.co.uk/matador
Twitter: @matadorbooks

ISBN 978 1800462 762

British Library Cataloguing in Publication Data.
A catalogue record for this book is available from the British Library.

Printed and bound in Great Britain by 4edge Limited
Typeset in 11pt Minion Pro by Troubador Publishing Ltd, Leicester, UK

Matador is an imprint of Troubador Publishing Ltd

To Mi Niña, without whose love, support, and patience, I would likely have not survived this experience.

To my family in general, who created the bond and the basis that has ever allowed me to find the return path to the surface after descending by morbid curiosity to the darkest chasms.

"Me gustas cuando callas porque estás como ausente"

("I like you when you are quiet because it is as though you are absent")

PABLO NERUDA

Contents

Once: Cocoon 1
   In the Beginning 3
   Cognitive Reserve 6
   The Road to Serfdom 12
   Though This Be Madness, Yet There Is Method in It 17
   Flies and Bugs on the Wall 21
   Phase Transition 26

Twice: Nemesis 31
   Lust for Life 33
   I Man a de Bush Doctor 37
   A Stumble Is Not a Fall 40
   Taxi Driver 43
   Daddy, Daddy! 48
   Conspiracy Nut 51
   Follow the Light 55

Thrice: Be Fruitful and Multiply, and Fill the Mind and Subdue It 59
   Peace after the Storm 61
   Mus 65
   Quousque Tandem Abutere, Mr Tantrum, Patienta Nostra? 69
   Counter-Strike 73
   Gasparín… 79
   … & Company 84

They're the Emotions, Stupid!	90
To Infinity, But Not Beyond	96
A Million Followers	100
That Dirty Little Coward That Shot Mr. Howard	104
We Shall Fight on the Beaches	108
The Nutty Professor	114
Lucy in the Sky with Diamonds	116
Business as Usual	121
Therapeutic Wanderings	124
Medicamentous Odyssey	129
It Takes One to Know One	135
Paradigm Shift	142
Fourth Time Lucky: Thou Shalt Never Get Rid of Us	145
On the Sands of Hesitation	147
One More Voice	150
The Rain in Spain Stays Mainly in the Plain	154
Freak Show (Again)	157
The Poverty of Socialism	161
People in Glass Houses Shouldn't Throw Stones	164
The Straw That Broke the Camel's Back	167
Journeys End in Lovers Meeting	171
Johnny, la Gente Está Muy Loca	175
Sixteen Tons	177
Take the Voices and Run	179
Réflexions Sur la Violence	181
Sitges Mon Amour	184
Growing Up. A Mountain Out of a Molehill	188
There Are More Things in Heaven and Earth, Horatio…	191
Sic Semper Tyrannis	195
Unvollendete	197

Introduction

Hearing voices is an uncanny, even scary, experience. It can be absurd, delusional, and grotesque. It can be comforting, too; some people hear, for a while, the voices of their loved ones who have recently passed away, and so they can say goodbye to them. For many, it is a symptom of insanity, but others find it harmless and estimable, perhaps esoteric. It is said that great characters in history, such as Joan of Arc, heard voices too. I have been hearing voices for a long time. I hardly recall what it is like to live without them. There are many different voices, dozens of voices, but I have never been able to count them.

Presently, all of them are male, but there have also been female ones. There is not a single moment at day or night in which there is not one or, more often, several of them speaking. I also hear them when dreaming. They always talk about my actions or thoughts, and, usually, though not always, they try to annoy me, make me jumpy, or even humiliate me.

Using the word 'hallucination' to name the phenomenon is an easy resource, but for those who do not know it, it is useless to describe the experience. A hallucination is an objectless perception, and, of course, these invisible bigmouths never appear anywhere. But the brain has evolved considering what it perceives to be real. My attempts to convince myself that I am not hearing anything are always in vain. It is not the case; I do hear them, and there is no way to avoid it; it does not depend on my will, they seem entirely alien, and those who speak are others.

There is nothing I can do to be certain that it is just something created out of nowhere inside my head. Moreover, my voices seem to come from outside my body. They are identical to actual people talking. They use many clichés and set phrases, but within ordinary speech; they do not use merely single phrases or words. The mind uses subterfuge to justify the presence of these unwanted intruders. It does so by producing beliefs. The oddest thing is that it does not seem bizarre to me. Physical impossibility is not a problem. It is not that I believe that someone may be talking to me from inside a lamp post; it is that my mind suspends judgement on the fact. I know it cannot happen, but I have no choice but to believe it is true. That sense of belief in something absurd is just one more intruder in my mind, one more hallucination. I cannot expel or neutralize it either. At most, I can ignore it.

Notwithstanding this, it is possible to keep in control and behave (almost) normally. I can live in two different worlds at the same time: a regular life in my relationships with those on the outside world while having fierce internal battles with invisible foes inside me. Only when this situation becomes overwhelming can one become a psychiatric patient.

In my case, there seems to be nothing to do to get rid of them. Antipsychotics are of little, if any, help. I have never met anyone who knew about any therapy for psychosis. The only advice I have been able to get from a psychiatrist about how to deal with the issue has been a cryptic: "Don't mind them". Good for psychiatry! It is like suggesting to a poor man that, to end his poverty, he has to make money. Perhaps it is a way of saying: "I'm sorry, but you are alone in this affair, you will have to get by on your own." Now I think this is the best option. You made your bed, and you lie in it.

All this happens in a world to which others do not have access, so I have to roll up my sleeves and learn to manage it. The voices try to take control, to master me. My decision has always been not to allow it in any way. I have combined that firm determination with categorical rejection through argumentation, but also with mockery, scorn, and wisecrack, which are much more effective weapons in the psychological field than anger.

Learning to manage conflict with no way out, but in which my physical integrity is not in danger – since nobody will break my nose if I cross the line – is an excellent school of life. I do not know what it is like to live with voices that support and advise you, as it happens to other people. Still, mine seem to have a strange fixation with dominating and trampling me in any way, and that is perhaps one of the worst approaches that one can choose when it comes to interacting with me. It is like a landing of rowdy Vikings, armed with an aggressive and tireless prattle, whom I can only neutralize but will never be able to throw back into the sea. The way of expressing each one gives me a precise insight into the kind of personality they have. They are usually pretty stereotypical characters. And they are stereotypes that are more than criticizable.

Aggressors, in the real world, are often dumb people. Their personalities are raw, barbaric, clumsy. The combination of aggressor and good people is inconceivable. This fact pretty much levels the conflict. No matter how many accusations they make to me, I can always accuse them of worse things. As though I had lived in a dangerous neighborhood, I have had to fight hard to get by. Over the years, I have been advancing, evolving, and adapting.

Personal growth is the best weapon for this kind of fight. Against the worst of society, I have learned to use the best of it. As my personality has been reinforced, I have learned to manage my emotions better and, with them, the problem. My inner world has become more civilized as I have civilized myself. "Don't mind them" is only the end of the story. It is up to me to write the rest.

My goal in writing this story is to provide testimony about hearing voices focused on the experience itself, rather than on the recovery process. This might be a rather unusual story, compared to those that I have read in other books. It is not the testimony of a psychiatric patient, but that of a slightly mental guy. For me, psychiatrists have had a role similar to that of the GP; virtually at no time have I been unable to control my life. I have doggedly searched here and there for some long story like this without success. I try and explain my life story in parallel, to put everything in context, but without too many details.

My life is not too exciting, nor is it exemplary. I am instead a first-hand witness to what goes on inside a person through whose mind almost all known psychiatric symptoms have passed. I would feel satisfied if someone finds any inspiration in my story, although I do not recommend anyone to try to imitate me.

I hope that nobody bothers if I often use a casual and even humorous tone. I do it only concerning my own story. I am very aware of the torture that this phenomenon can constitute for many people. For me, it often has been. I have read terrible stories of abuse and all kinds of trauma before the appearance of the voices. It is not a joke at all, but a sense of humour has helped me a great deal in my battle; I cannot do without it when it comes to relating my own experience.

This is a story without names. Only a few voices will have a name, the nickname I have given them. I will not mention the name of any real person in the story; at most, I will use their initials. I will refer to my wife only with the sobriquets that I usually use with her: '*Mi Niña*' or '*Bonita*'. I am just Miguel. Miguel with no more; '*a secas*', as we say in Spanish – without surnames, as the voices call me.

Once: Cocoon

In the Beginning

This story begins like many other stories of psychosis, paranoia, and delusions: with frequent drug use that raises until it becomes abuse. This was gradually short-circuiting more and more mental mechanisms, distorting the perception of reality, and adding to the actual world several elements that are not really there.

But this is not a story about drug abuse, with parties, messing around, hangovers, mental gaps, and so on. There are already hundreds of those stories, and there is no longer anything very original to say about all of that. It is a world that amazes no one anymore. I would have to go far back in time and talk about too many irrelevant things. I will only say that I had tried, over many years, a vast range of legal and illegal products in a relentless quest for extreme sensations. Given that, let us start at a convenient point of time.

This point is the year 1994. At that time, I was twenty-nine. The fact that marks the beginning of the story is something as ordinary as a move. My girlfriend and I were renting an apartment in the Lavapiés neighborhood in Madrid; our first home. The owner of the house needed it for her son, so she did not renew our agreement and we had to go. We found a fantastic apartment in Pelayo Street, in the Chueca neighborhood, next to the General Society of Authors and Editors.

It was on the fourth floor, the only flat on the top floor, and there was no lift, but we were young, and we were not afraid to climb stairs. It had three rooms, the first of them without windows. The living room and the second one, which would be my workroom, overlooked Pelayo Street; the kitchen and the third one, the bedroom, overlooked a '*corrala*' patio, around which were distributed the interior dwellings of the building. A large dinette compensated for the small kitchen. The bathroom, located between the kitchen and the bedroom, was pretty and bright, and its window also overlooked the patio. The apartment was rented empty, unfurnished. Rental prices had dropped and we would be paying less than before for a larger apartment. All seemed perfect.

We owned just a bed, some office furniture, the TV set and little else, for the previous apartment was semi-furnished. We were not made of money, but there was no problem. At night, Madrid's sidewalks are full of discarded old furniture, some in good condition. There is always some rubbish bin around. These bins are the perfect place to dispose of bulky items when no one is looking. We walked the streets looking for chairs, tables, sideboards… anything we could carry since we did not have a car. Discovering useful things in rubbish became almost an obsession.

We were also given old furniture from our friends and relatives. We bought a couple of wardrobes, the cheapest ones, and put them in the interior room, which became the 'closet' room. The house looked like a furniture showroom. No chair was the same as any other, the sofa was uncomfortable, and the television was on the floor. IKEA did not yet exist in Madrid at that time.

I work, and I was working then, with computers. I am a software developer. At that time, I was self-employed, and I worked at home. I am a very independent guy. I like people, but I also like being alone. One has to know how to manage both things: I prefer to be with people to have fun and for leisure, but to be alone to work. And so I had managed to make it.

I worked for a small company located in an apartment in the Salamanca neighborhood. They were unusual people, some of the best I have ever met. The bosses were a lovely couple, and the employees were all peculiar in some way. My brother had finished his physics degree. He worked setting up concert stages, something that was also physical, but that was not his thing. I managed, without much effort, to get him hired as well. In addition to physics, he also knew how to write software. Guaranteed work.

There was someone else who lived with us too, whom I have yet to introduce. His name was '*Gato*' and, as it is not very difficult to guess, he was a cat. Specifically, a black cat. A cat picked up from the street where we lived in our old apartment – the king of the house.

All this constitutes the normal part of the matter. Now it is time to include the drugs.

Upon arriving at the new house, I was in a more or less calm stage where the excesses were limited to little more than alcohol consumption on weekends. I missed something stronger, but I did not want it to be too much. So, one day, I reviewed my mental vade mecum, and I recalled a particular substance. It was methylphenidate, abbreviated as d-MPH, related to amphetamines. It is much easier to get from pharmacies because it is less potent. Madrid is full of pharmacies; there must be thousands. In the eighties, almost as many drugs came out of pharmacies as from pushers' pockets.

That time was over now, but one could still get a little something. I had to walk the streets a lot. It was impossible to get anything in many of the pharmacies, but eventually the quest always ended up paying off. I will skip the fact that I used these tablets recreationally on weekends, to focus on a much more severe and beginner's mistake: I started using them at work, too.

This meant I started to take them every day and ended up doing it at all hours. The process has no interest: you start taking a few and end up taking many. As with tobacco, you reach a peak and then stay there. My peak became thirty tablets a day, a whole box. Every day of the week, every week of the year. It was the first thing I did when I got up and the last before going to bed. As happens to coffee addicts, stimulants, in the end, also help sleep.

To regulate so much stimulation, I had also to consume something relaxing, and I resorted to chemistry. The most common option for that is benzodiazepines, but I chose codeine, for it was easy to get without a prescription. I also took a little every day. I divided my daily routine between working, long walks to visit pharmacies, and some sporadic visits to the office. And, of course, chronic drug consumption. No wonder something was concocting inside me.

Cognitive Reserve

There is an explanation for the fact that the same brain disorders do not affect everyone the same way. Some people completely lose control and the link with reality; others are disabled to different degrees. Some, as in my case, can even lead a more or less normal life. The reason is known as 'cognitive reserve'.

Many complex systems, made up of a myriad of interconnected, interactive components, are arranged as a network. Specifically, they present an architecture which is 'scale-free'. The elements that make up a network are the nodes – people, cities, neurons – and the links between them are relationships, roads, synapses. In the scale-free networks, there are many nodes with few links and few nodes highly connected. The name 'scale-free' means that if you count all the nodes that have any number of connections, there are always many more nodes that have fewer.

A significant property of these networks is that they are very robust to aleatory failures. It is possible to randomly remove many nodes before the web is too affected, with completely disconnected areas. The Internet, for example, is organized this way. Initially, it was a network for military use designed in the USA during the Cold War. The goal was that, in the face of a nuclear attack by the Communist bloc, the network would continue connecting the country even if partially destroyed. When a road is closed due to works, there is always an alternative way to reach our destination. The road network also follows this architecture. These networks, however, are susceptible to the destruction of highly connected nodes. Removal of nodes of this type quickly disconnects the net, which gets divided into several isolated subnets.

The organization of neural networks is scale-free too. There are billions of neurons – nodes – in the brain, which are interconnected by a hundred trillion synapses. Researchers have performed post-mortem studies comparing brains with a similar degree of deterioration. Some of the subjects had developed pathologies, such as the fearsome Alzheimer's disease. However, others had no remarkable sign of disorder when they died. Thus, the cognitive reserve consists of what remains in good condition in the brain after an injury or other type of failure has occurred, whether or not it is reversible.

Thinking of the brain as a simple homogeneous network of interconnected neurons is an overly simplistic model. There are different types of neurons specialized in various tasks, and they are not all alike. In synapses, there are some substances called neurotransmitters. They determine the effect that each of the connections has on the neurons on which they act. This effect can be of two types: excitatory or inhibitory. If it is excitatory, the neuron that receives the discharge is activated and discharges in turn, through its synapses, neurotransmitters on neighboring neurons. If the effect is inhibitory, the opposite happens. The same neuron receives connections from many others and also connects to a more or less high number of neighbors.

Therefore, the neuron can receive both inhibitory and excitatory impulses. The average of these effects determines the final action of the neuron. It also determines the speed and intensity of the response. Furthermore, there are several different neurotransmitters, with varied effects on our moods and emotions. Furthermore, synapses, the connections between neurons, can be more or less strong. Their strength changes over time: the cell can create, reinforce, weaken, or reabsorb them depending on their activity. The response rate of the neuron can also vary, for the transmission of the impulse depends on the entrance and exit of electrically charged particles, named 'ions', through the cell membrane. For this task, there are many pores, called 'ion channels', that the cell can also create and reabsorb. Those mechanisms are the basis of learning and of the imbalances that can occur in our brain. The amount of possibilities makes one dizzy.

Reducing the study to the neurons and their connections, complex as it may be, is insufficient. Neurons form specialized subnets, with few or thousands of cells. These subnets group into larger pools: subnet networks.

These aggregates are also interconnected, even with other aggregates located in quite distant areas of the brain. This way, the cerebrum is made up of clearly differentiable parts, such as the hippocampus, the amygdala, or the cerebellum. The types of neurons that predominate in them are different, as are the tasks for which they are responsible. Even within one of these parts, there can be different areas that are activated or deactivated when we perform various activities, such as talking, reading, or jumping.

Not only brain activity is relevant. The inhibition, that is, inactivity, is also essential. For everything to work properly, some areas must be silent, so we can say that the whole brain participates in any activity we do or anything we feel or perceive. Thus, some parts have to be silent for us to function normally, and they keep quiet because other parts order it.

All this balance, albeit extremely complex, is quite robust. Despite the malfunction of some elements, others try to override the failure taking control. However, it is impossible to prevent the accumulation of imbalances from leading to an altered mental condition from which it may be impossible to get out. The brain goes from a convenient state of equilibrium to an inconvenient one. There is no need for injury. It is enough that the neurons rearrange in a problematic way through the natural mechanisms of learning and forgetting.

Some imbalances are more or less easy to solve. The lack or excess of any neurotransmitter can be compensated using drugs. Drugs, however, are a very rough approximation for a problem derived from neuronal disorganization. They can stop the atypical behavior of neurons, but recomposing the connections is another matter; to achieve that, therapy is usually essential.

The brain is responsible for centralizing the operation of the body; it receives chemical signals from the rest of the organs, in the form of hormones and other compounds. The cerebrum sends back other signals to perform essential functions such as breathing or heartbeat. However, these mechanisms are insufficient to interact with a complex and changing external environment. We also need to interact with other species of living beings, especially with other humans. To make this possible, a large part of our brain has specialized in generating the conscious. The conscious self is a kind of leader in charge of guiding the organism. It has the five senses to perceive the external environment; it also has proprioception, a sort of sense directed towards the interior of the body that allows it to know its state. The self processes all this information in the form of sensations, thrills, feelings, or reason, depending on its complexity. All these states give back information to the lower levels of the organism, which generates a feedback cycle that allows the survival of the whole. We are not the goal of evolution; we are just a result of it.

The self is actually part of a broader community of organic mechanisms, built by a community of cells, which are themselves formed by another community of genes, simple organic molecules made up of billions of atoms of only five different elements: carbon, nitrogen, oxygen, hydrogen and phosphorous.

All of this activity continually shapes our brains. Connections are formed and destroyed; ion channels are created and reabsorbed. The structures that remain in time give rise to what we call memory. There is a simplistic view of memory as 'something' that is 'somewhere' in the brain and where we store mysterious things we refer to as 'memories'. Nevertheless, memory is nothing more than a set of all active and functional synapses in our brain. We can use several criteria to classify the activity of different neurons and neural networks, as well as their effect; likewise, we can consider that there exist different types of memory.

Various mechanisms, spread throughout the brain, can act with different intensity so that the learned remains, reinforces or weakens. So it is possible that some damage or disorder affects one 'type' of memory more than another, or that we forgot certain things as the connections between the areas that house these synapses and other regions of the brain deteriorate. Recalling is the reverse activation of this recording mechanism: reproducing the recorded sensations. Memory is not only nourished by reality. It can be arduous to know and understand reality. Human beings have a powerful device that allows us to make hypotheses to generate a kind of tentative knowledge about reality. Science relies on this ability. Evolution has endowed us with a mechanism that helps us to consider a priori any more or less plausible hypothesis, the sensation or emotion called 'belief', which in its extreme version is called 'certainty'.

Indeed, we can convert beliefs into certainties without too much effort. We can make fantastic hypotheses about things whose existence or possibility is not even possible to verify. We can devise imaginary characters, know that they are fictitious, and still consider possible their existence, find them credible.

Everything that circulates through our brain, be it real or imaginary, can be added to memory. The act of recording and that of reproducing the recorded are different, although both generate similar mental states. In general, they are voluntary acts, so we know how to distinguish a given experience from its memory. But memories are not just static photographs. Nature is inherently dynamic, processes that are in motion and change. Our mind is adapted to that. It is capable of reconstructing very complex dynamic processes, perhaps the most complex of which is to rebuild mentally another person.

It is said that 'we learn the others', and this is quite a wise sentence. We learn the characteristic expressions, the way to move, to speak, to show emotions… from the people we meet. We add other features that we hypothetically presume. We can also add traits that they do not have at all, to praise or denigrate them. And we can believe that these devised characteristics are real ones. We can say that this knowledge is induced by other people in our brain, as though they used our neurons to create an image of themselves in our minds. They are conscious and intelligent agents, they can do it, and it is called 'manipulation'. Even smart animals know how to do it.

Thereby we can build simulacra of unknown people using known features. We call these mocks 'stereotypes', and they can be as credible as the mental avatars of actual people we know. They can also represent all members of a collective. We can build fictional characters in our minds, create them through what we read in a book, or even put a personalized voice on them.

When our brain works with normality, which is a very complex state with fuzzy margins, we know how to distinguish between reality and fiction quite well (at least according to the official version). We also recognize if what appears in our mind is produced by our will or is induced from outside. Further, we all have access to a naturally altered state of mind: dreams. In dreams, these replicants, learned or created in the waking state, come to life and present themselves to us as actual people.

We know, or we are pretty sure, that dreams are something produced by our mental activity. But the mechanisms that make us aware of that in a waking state seem to be disconnected during sleep. If we dream about our brother, he is truly our brother, not a fake character, nor does it seem a memory of our brother. When he speaks to us, our brother is speaking to us in person; we do not perceive his speech as if we were making up what he says. If a dreamed killer is chasing us, he looks like a real killer. It is a stranger, but an actual stranger. The fear it produces is also a real fear. When we are killed in a dream, we suddenly wake up. Luckily, our minds do not know what it is like to die. Anyway, we feel the need to escape.

With all these elements, we can now reconstruct any mental disorder for anyone who has never had it. It is made up of mental states produced by an excess or defect of neuronal activity, by 'incorrect' interactions among neural networks. There are exaggerated or absurd beliefs and other emotions; some may be lacking; they arise in us hallucinations generated by them or that support them. Brain development, especially in childhood stages, can be altered by a multitude of factors, both internal and external. Neural networks interconnect depending on what happens to us in life and the emotions it produces. All these processes run based on fixed patterns that make us seem alike in substance.

Merely with our usual thinking and behavior, we can cause ourselves mental disorders: obsessions, depressive states, or addictions such as gambling. We learn to develop them, and they remain recorded; later, it is challenging to stop playing them back. Nonetheless, these disorders may be only partial. One can be pathologically jealous of a partner's friends but have normal behavior with other people.

In the most severe manifestation of psychosis, schizophrenia, control is almost completely lost, and one plunges into a world dominated by delusions and hallucinations. I have been an exceptional witness to many of these altered states. I have experienced them in the first person, and I have retained enough sanity to be able to observe and analyze them firsthand. The mind and its nature have always fascinated me. So I have never doubted taking advantage of the opportunity that has been presented to me and making the best of it. Based on my many years of experience, I have been able to come up with some hypotheses of my own. Those hypotheses, of course, might not be correct.

The Road to Serfdom

Many people think that having psychosis means to be entirely out of touch with reality and that it is something that happens more or less suddenly. However, this disorder is a progressive process in which small distortions of perception accumulate, and delusional ideas are built with a certain logic. Rationalism has led us to think in logic and reason as opposed to, or at least complementary to, feelings and emotions. Notwithstanding, if you carefully examine everything that happens in your mind, you will end up finding that there is nothing other than sensations, emotions, and feelings.

A mental image of a tree or a rock is made up of sensations. Feelings of fear or joy are emotions, but a belief, certainty, or conclusion are emotions too. Nature is elegant, for it gives rise to immense complexity with a few simple elements. Reason is just the most sophisticated bunch of thrills we have, the subtler, finest-grained ones. Mathematical logic is no more than a simplified model of the natural one that rules our mind, which works hand in hand with the rest of our emotions.

The environment and circumstances can make notable contributions to distorting ideas. If this distortion lingers and increases, the usual dynamic of some mental processes changes and reveals the disorder, which can become permanent. Physicists name it 'phase transition'. The process intensifies if a combination of several factors occurs. Smoking is harmful; smoking and drinking alcohol is worse; smoking, drinking alcohol, and little sleep is even worse, and so on, until your body says 'enough', and you get sick. It seems that the disorder appears suddenly, but it is the result of a silent and progressive fight in which several defense mechanisms struggle with the external aggressions, trying to stabilize the organism functions until the damage is too severe. The breakthrough takes place, which triggers the catastrophe.

Back to the story… the company for which I was working produced multimedia applications, very popular at that time. We used to record something like a magazine, an encyclopedia, or a course on CDs. The format was similar to what one would find online nowadays on a website: images, sounds, special effects, links and so on. My specialty was writing this kind of code. One day, one of those projects, more ambitious than usual, came up. It was about developing an editor to quickly design and build multimedia applications without having to be a developer. One just had to place the texts, photos, sounds, etc., using the mouse, indicating when and with what effects each item should appear. In the early nineties, you had to do almost all the work yourself, from scratch.

I started designing the whole thing in great detail. My head was boiling with ideas about sophisticated and complex systems. The truth is that I did not develop a simple and straightforward approach, but rather a kind of gobbledygook, a rigmarole. The name I gave it speaks for itself: 'Aleph', the letter of the Hebrew alphabet with which the mathematicians designate the different degrees of infinity. I was then already taking some occasional d-MPH tablets, the same as others drink coffee. They did not get me very high, as amphetamines or cocaine can do, but it did make me more enthusiastic than was normal.

The time came to present the design, and I met with P, the company director, and a great person, who also had great ideas that were often overenthusiastic, too. Another developer who had recently joined the company attended the meeting. He was one of the good ones, which meant that it was almost impossible to discuss his way of making software. He was very clear that things should be done his way. The same could be said about me, and, unfortunately, his way of seeing the project was completely different from mine: it was more straightforward and more realistic. It seemed to him that I was daydreaming. For me, his vision was too limited. We started a discussion that couldn't have an end; he was very calm and I got more and more excited – with the help of chemistry – albeit without raising my voice and shouting. Instead, I was devoured by angst caused by his misunderstanding of something that to me was so obvious.

At some point, the boss got fed up and stopped the sterile argument we were having: I would do what I had in mind with the editor, and my colleague was assigned to another part of the project. I left the office in such a state of nerves that it was mentioned many times after the incident. The poor fellow, somewhat unfairly, got the reputation of being obdurate, and was almost blamed for driving me crazy. This event, I think, was the first sign that things were starting to go wrong in my head.

It happens to many software developers, especially at the beginning of our careers – causing despair to our bosses – that we can see so clearly what we have to do that we think it will take much less time than necessary. We focus on our ideal world and do not take into account the unforeseen events. Over time, those who ask us by when we are going to finish learn to interpret 'two days' as two weeks and 'one month' as a quarter of a year. In principle, it becomes a disadvantage in terms of credibility. With experience and the passing of time, it becomes an advantage: when it finally takes two days to finish what you intended to finish in two days, your bosses still think that it will take you a week, just in case. Then, you go from working against the clock to doing the job more calmly and feeling more relaxed.

Unfortunately, at that point I had not yet reached that level. The number of tablets I was taking was increasing. I had the bad habit of categorically stating that I would soon have something to show. And I honestly believed it. Only I was wrong. My boss scheduled again and again meetings with potential customers to present our brand-new product to them. On my side, there were sleepless nights the days before those meetings. There were days when I almost had something to show; almost, but not quite. Then, more pills to keep working, more stress, and more pressure upon my back. Frustration the day of the meeting, shambling back home defeated, to collapse in bed. P, trying to deal with the potential customers as best as possible. A, my boss's wife, who ran the company administration, often repeated that if I continued like this, the situation would end up in a *surmenage* (a kind of nervous breakdown along with a chronic state of fatigue). Things were going astray, but this was not going to be the outcome.

When one occasionally works under the influence of stimulants, one can make substantial advances very fast. When one does it all the time, something like running on a treadmill or exercise bike occurs. It does not matter the energy and the effort put into it; one is forever in the same place.

I wrote the program code like a possessed man. Ideas flowed in my mind as the alcohol flows at a college fraternity party hosted by John Belushi. Hundreds, thousands of lines of code written obsessively. That was a piece of cake. I had in my mind clearly designed the whole application. I just had to get it out of there and transfer it to the computer. It was an epiphany, a glorious moment of enlightenment, a kind of silent Mozart orchestrating a soundless symphony with my computer keyboard. I was a maven, a virtuoso.

Glory has its counterpoint in hell, and my moments of creative illumination had it in the compilation inferno. Compiling is the operation of finding code syntax errors and, if they do not exist, converting the code into an executable program. I wrote thousands of lines of code before compiling, and each one had several errors, so compilation ended up being an endless loop. There was no way to check whether the program was working as intended. There was always something wrong. While correcting the mistakes, new ideas popped up that I enthusiastically caught, adding new errors to the code. It is not that I was going around in a circle; I was immersed in a chaotic attractor. I was going through similar states over and over, without ever repeating them in the same way, so it was even trickier to get out of the situation.

The manic state was not restricted to programming. I ended up being unable to carry on many other activities. Bringing any object from my workroom to the kitchen became a never-ending tour through the whole apartment. I would begin countless simultaneous tasks that popped into my mind along the way. Everything was suggesting something else to do or to relocate, and I usually ended up laden with a multitude of junk in a pathetic attempt to optimize, which would transform into a dead-end trap.

My social life declined hugely until it virtually disappeared. Getting out turned into a feat. I always would have to finish something beforehand. Going out to have a drink over the weekend could start at 10 p.m. with a "Wait, I'm almost done" and ending at 4 a.m. with a "Leave it, let's go to bed". It was impossible to get to an appointment on time (if I even went). The notion of time was completely blurred. Hours could go by in what seemed like minutes to me. My activity was frantic and obsessive.

I felt compelled to undertake everything I could think of to do, no matter how irrelevant. It was the embodiment of the myth of Sisyphus, only with many more stones. I spent hours, days, and many nights sitting at the computer, writing lines, and more lines of sterile code. It was like a curse, trapped by my own emotions, without escape.

My insight into the environment also began to change little by little. Things were still there, but I no longer felt them as usual. With perception and proprioception altered, I was on the threshold of psychosis. I found myself at the tipping point between altered mood and altered real-world interpretation. I started having these feelings of alienation during the holidays in a camping place in Rosas, in the province of Gerona. The things I saw looked normal, but the feeling of seeing them was slightly different. I heard the voices of people speaking around me, but the sensation that came from hearing them was not the same as usual. While I didn't quite know how to explain what was changing, I knew there was something that was doing it.

It might appear that this would be more than enough reason to panic and *ipso facto* stop consuming the stimulant tablets or whatever I was taking. Mightn't it? Well, it didn't. I just had to control it a bit; maybe I was crossing the line. Take it easy, man. Most smokers continue smoking, even knowing that they can inflict serious health problems; even after a heart attack. Logic is not a great counsellor for an addict. The winner of the battle among all our internal desires leads the will. It takes the same willpower to quit smoking as it does to continue smoking against the odds. The key is to direct it to the most advisable address, though we usually do it to the one that is the least effort. It is natural, we have to save energy, but it is a saving that sometimes ends up taking its toll on us.

I don't know for sure how long I maintained this lifestyle, but it was months, at least. I remember thinking, shortly before all this happened, that life was too dull and that I would like to live in a fantasy world where I could find a dragon around the corner. Ask, and ye shall receive. Intense experiences were brewing.

Though This Be Madness, Yet There Is Method in It

With emotions, perception, and interpretation of reality altered, plus a constant supply of triggering factors, I was bound to have a psychotic breakdown sooner or later. However, I developed this outbreak methodically, following specific schemes. In cases of abusive consumption of toxic substances, it is not strange to develop feelings of guilt. As much as I tried to ignore it, I knew that my health was in danger. It was also frowned upon socially. One may also be unable to fulfill obligations, causing detriment to others. It is a kind of defense mechanism that tries to counteract the impulses that move you to stick to your guns. Feelings of guilt brought up the idea that I was going to get caught, that others were going to realize the real causes of my state, and I started to be careful and vigilant to avoid it.

I used to snort the d-MPH tablets, crushing first and then inhaling them to speed up the effect. I was afraid that people could see traces of white powder on my nose, so I began to avoid looking at others in the face. I always looked elsewhere while talking to someone, which increased my stress. It is exhausting to be so alert to everything you do. When one tries to act naturally, the result is just to act more weirdly – as one makes these unusual behaviors more and more frequently. And I realized it, but I kept doing it.

One day, like almost every day, I had gone out in the morning to roam pharmacies to buy more tablets. I had become used to carefully observe the environment, just in case I came across some acquaintance. That day I realized that my fears were not unfounded; my co-worker JP was following me from across the street. I didn't think it was a hallucination. There was definitely someone who was, or so it seemed to me, identical to JP. As I was close to my parents' home, I thought that the most natural thing was to say hello, as usual, and tell him that I was there to visit my relatives. When the doppelgänger saw that I was heading towards him, he turned back and quickly walked away. He was spooked, for sure. My appearance was not that of a nice guy; I was becoming quite wan and thin. He must have figured I meant to rob him or something. Anyhow, this confirmed my suspicions; they were following me, and they didn't want me to find out.

This conclusion induced in me a mix of fear and satisfaction. I was in trouble, but at least I knew I was. Then it was time to give the affair a coherent and convincing explanation. Regular people's logic often leaves much to be desired. We all misunderstand some situations and attitudes, but deranged people's logic can be like a magician's top hat; anything can get out from there. The two of us were quite far from the office. It was during my colleague's working hours. Unlike me, he was an employee; he was off-site. Therefore, there had to be more people involved. The bosses had to also be in on it. It might seem absurd to think that these people, who were just my colleagues, could conspire to do something like that, but that was not a problem. I quickly built an explanation to fit my expectations, my fears. The so-called 'confirmation bias' is an ancestral survival trait. Usually, it is better to get a non-existent danger wrong than ignoring a real one.

Common sense had not completely gone. On the one hand, I was almost convinced of the conspiracy. At the same time, I had strong doubts about the possibility of something like that. Two opposite criteria to explain the same reality, neither of which could impose on the other. I needed material evidence that what I suspected was actually happening. Other people might have rushed and made a scene. They would also have ended up before the psychiatrist, if not straight in the booby hatch. I needed more evidence and, of course, complete leeway. Nor did I seem to be very clear on what to do in such a case, so I decided to continue investigating and behave as if I suspected nothing.

The most logical thing was to go straight to the office with any excuse to check if my chap was there. If he had gone home to change his clothes, I would arrive first; if not, he would be dressed as I had seen him minutes ago.

'Elementary, my dear Watson.' A conspiracy can only be uncovered if one pays attention to even the smallest details. So I took the Metro right then and there and, a few stops later, I reached my goal, the office, with the excuse that I had to copy some files.

No one seemed surprised, of course. JP was there. Somehow he had managed to change his clothes. Maybe he'd had them ready in the office, and he hadn't had to stop at home. After all, it was a conspiracy. They should have planned events like that. He also did not seem surprised to see me, nor did he appear nervous about the incident. He acted as if nothing had happened, with total normality.

At first, it had seemed to me that I would get much more conclusive, even irrefutable, evidence. Now, the results of my cunning move reinforced both the attorney's and the prosecutor's arguments. The attitude I perceived was both guilty concealment and a sign of my mistake. It was necessary to continue investigating. After all, I had seen him with my very own eyes. 'Absence of evidence is not evidence of absence.' This is the paranoid curse.

I started dropping round more often to the office to find out if the spying I suspected existed; I even started trying to listen to the conversations sneakily. Not having a desk assigned, I settled in a meeting room, where I was alone. The perfect situation for others to blabber on me, thinking I wouldn't hear them. I was beginning to be the center of the universe.

I suppose that everyone has sometimes thought they have heard a melody over some repeating, monotonous sound, such as the vibration of an engine. Eventually, the motor seems to end up 'playing' the tune we want. There is a game the name of which I do not know: You whisper something in the ear of a playmate; he re-whispers it to another person, and so on. The last one in the chain says out loud what he has understood, which is then compared with the original message. It is quite difficult to understand what people say in other rooms, especially without knowing who is talking to whom or if they are on the phone. The brain has a natural mechanism to fill in the gaps left by imperfect perception, to create provisional sensory illusions that help us to catch reality, no matter one has to correct it later. If you shuffle all the letters in a text, except the first and the last of each word, you can nevertheless still read and understand it entirely. When we listen to someone talking in a language that is little known to us, we usually complete the sentences, once uttered, with the words that we have not fully understood, to give them an appropriate meaning according to the context.

Something like this happened with my listening business. At last, I ended up deciphering all sorts of evidence, the confirmation bias mentioned above, by which one always gives more relevance to whatever information supports the opinion already formed. At the same time, there was no way to convince me fully. Each time, I pondered that I could be wrong, that everything could be a misunderstanding. After all, I could hardly grasp what people said. I had surmised most of their words, so what I thought I had understood could not have been uttered. I didn't know then, but I was incubating the voices.

The finding and collecting of evidence was not the only research that I was carrying out. I had to build a case, find a motive, discover all those involved, and what their different roles were. The truth is that I did not feel threatened at all, just annoyed. What they were doing was, ultimately, for my sake, not to hurt me. They were concerned about my health; in fact, more worried than I was. It could be an annoying proceeding, but in no way did it arouse feelings of aggressiveness in me. I was trying to figure out how to escape the situation. It seemed to me that it was a kind of unconscious defense mechanism to avoid the damage that I was consciously causing my body. Everyone circling around me and my harmful activities. Everything focused on the problem.

The purpose of the conspiracy could not be other than to section me. But for that, 'they' would have to bring the case to court after a doctor had requested it. The knowledge that I believed to have about this procedure came from movies, news, novels, and other media. Still, it was not too far from reality; to be admitted, I had to present out-of-control behavior, which was not, and was not going to be, the case, and my relatives should have requested it. My brother was already working at the company, and he had the keys to my apartment, so it was obviously one of them. My father, as an ascent relative, would be in charge of requesting admission. My boss, directly harmed and with the means and staff, in addition to having regular contact with me, was the organizer of the operation. I was facing a dilemma; I had to prove whether this was all true or false. With the script already drawn up, the play could begin. The actors could be set in motion.

Flies and Bugs on the Wall

Too many efforts to unravel the conspiracy that was being hatched around me. Too much concentration to decipher until the very last word had been uttered. All of that mixed with the effects of so many stimulants and stress. The areas of the brain that deal with language became highly sensitive; they started to work on their own and out of time. It was no longer necessary for people to be present for me to hear them talking. The first auditory hallucinations occurred: the voices.

There was a slight difference between illusions – when trying to understand the words of a voice I was really hearing – and hallucinations. Hallucinations were less confusing, for there was no interference with what was actually being said. Other than that, auditory hallucinations seem identical to the voices of real people. In the case that they belong to known people, they have their same tone of voice, use their characteristic expressions, and convey their same personality. Except for the strange behavior of spying on me, it was as if they were them. Details such as the fact that I could hear them clearly, even if they were a long way away, were irrelevant since the remainder qualities seemed one hundred per cent credible. As in a trial, evidence for and against the deeds was presented to my mind. The senses have an enormous weight in our interpretation of reality. Logic weighs considerably less.

If one is also willing to believe in the unlikely, or even the impossible, common sense has no chance of winning. For instance, one argument in favor was that I could easily understand what they were saying at a distance because they were well known people to me. The ear can be trained to do this. Do you need a supporting explanation? Isn't it true that in overloud environments, such as in a factory, workers can listen to and understand one another because they have become used to filtering noise? Paraphrasing Groucho Marx: 'These are my reasons. If you do not like them, I have others.' One reason is always found. If one is determined to corroborate or deny something, you will end up doing it. Even though the only person convinced is yourself.

In this way, the hints favoring the possibility or truth of what I was hearing were accumulating. Furthermore, the use of cameras and microphones was usual in the company, and these devices were frequently mentioned. The word 'recording' was often uttered. They would make recordings, they would watch recordings, and they would discuss the contents of the damn recordings. Having the key to my home, they could access whatever they wanted to bug. That was the reason why they could comment on what I was doing at home. I, in turn, could hear their comments while they spied on me from the street, within the radius of action of the devices. Close, but always hidden where I could not see them.

It was absurd: why do you hide if you don't care that I can hear you? It was unclear whether they realized I could hear them. Anyway, sometimes we hear from our homes people talking on the street or neighbors in their homes. Sometimes we even understand almost everything they say. I began to pay attention to this detail, to pay attention to everyone who was talking on the street, trying to find out how far I could understand what people were saying. I could also hear them speaking on the stairs, perhaps on the landing below mine, out of sight. But they were never there when I looked. I was convinced that the whole thing was real, while determined to prove that it was not the case; maybe to escape from what was an overwhelming reality. If they were just hallucinations, there was nothing to worry about, nothing was happening. It was the world upside down, the mechanism of evasion of reality when it becomes uncomfortable, working to return me to it.

There was another factor that facilitated my father's performance in the plot: there was a neighbor in the block whose voice was identical or very similar to his. Or, at least, that's what it seemed to me. Occasionally he could be heard saying something loud enough. Whatever he said had no real importance but I would give it meaning. Once into the intrigue, my mind had already learned to make it appear out of nowhere by creating his corresponding avatar. In this first phase, the voices used to talk about me and to one another, but not to me. They always seemed more obsessed with me than I was with them. My father was even, from time to time, accompanied by a psychiatrist to discuss my actions and the possibility of sectioning me.

Cameras and microphones are real objects. It seems very easy to prove whether they are actually there just by finding them. The problem was that I would only have real evidence if I actually found them. Again, the absence of evidence is not evidence of absence. If I couldn't find them, they were better hidden than I had thought. The first thing one should try to do is locate them. I thought that tiny cameras didn't exist at that time or, if they did, their price was too high. But things like that used to appear in the movies: flexible cameras that went through holes or crannies; tiny microphones inside sockets, under tables, in drawers, in lamps, in the most unexpected places. That was enough evidence for me; technological spying was possible. So I searched all over the house for these devices over and over again. With no success, of course.

The cameras seemed the easiest thing to find, as they needed to be at least in part visible for them to be useful. It was easy to know for sure where they were not. A bare wall, for example, cannot host a camera. I tried to figure out blind spots, listening to what the voices were saying about my activity. None of the furniture escaped scrutiny. Of course, nothing appeared anywhere. In the interior room, on top of the cabinets, there was a pile of junk – I am prone to keep everything. I checked everywhere very carefully. There had to be something hidden. That was the only way they could see me when I locked myself in there. But I found nothing, not even a trace of cameras. There was a suspicious item in the middle of the ceiling – the end of a piece of tube through which to pass cables. I lived on the top floor and there was an attic with access to the roof above my apartment. The door to that attic was located just above my front door. It was locked with a padlock, for which I had the key – and therefore, 'they' had, too.

The truth is that I never got in there. I only looked inside from the door, without seeing anything unusual. There seemed to be nothing and nobody there. But how could I know what was happening when I didn't look? Nowadays, with lots of cheap technology, I would have set up a broad counter-surveillance device for sure. But the price then was astronomical. Also, I did not live alone. What excuses would I give to Mi Niña? And how would I hoax my watchers into catching them by surprise? No matter which way I looked at it, I couldn't see a way to set up successful counter-intelligence.

I did all that searching, of course, while I was alone at home on weekdays. Bonita worked in the same company as my father; he was her boss. She did not know anything. I didn't tell her either. I tried to act with normality in front of everyone else, even in front of those who, supposedly, were conspiring to lock me up. Bonita was not part of the conspiracy. The inclusion of characters seemed to be fairly selective. In my case, female voices seldom came up. My mother appeared only once, and it was to recriminate the others for what they were doing.

Although I used to take it bravely, I also had low periods in which I cried like a baby. Crying helps in releasing stress. The intake of stimulants, together with lack of sleep, also causes depressive stages. I never became desperate, but I was quite distressed. Though the voices were relentless, they never enraged me. My boss's wife, A, who was also a lawyer, used to reprehend them from time to time. What they were doing didn't seem right to her. Besides being cruel, it was useless. One cannot achieve legitimate objectives using illegal means. But nothing could be done, all of them were doggedly sticking to the job in hand. Meanwhile, I continued to deliberate between fully believing and totally rejecting the whole thing.

While finding the cameras proved impossible, at least I thought I should be able to find the mics. I'm quite used to talking to myself, sometimes even loudly, albeit in a low tone, almost whispering. The voices could listen to even that, so there definitely were microphones somewhere. And they were good ones.

The problem was that this could require completely taking apart the flat. In the hours that I sometimes spent in the office, it was quite usual to notice the absence of one of my workmates, including my brother. In that company, one could go out for a walk to stretch one's legs. Of course, I suspected they were going to my home to lay their devices and collect the recordings. What was I going to do? I had decided to act normally so I could neither refuse to go to the office when necessary nor leave suddenly with no reason, to try to catch them red-handed, with the smoking gun. Also, it would have been useless; someone would have phoned them from the office (to my home, as then we didn't yet have mobile phones).

One day I almost lost my temper. Back then, the Internet was still a novelty. There were no social networks, but our email boxes were full of links or attached videos that friends and acquaintances often sent us. In the office, my co-workers spent all day showing videos to one another. Many of them contained pornographic scenes. That day they were watching and commenting on one in which a woman was in the shower. I thought that they were talking about one of their recordings, in which the woman who appeared taking a shower was no other than Mi Niña. They had crossed the line. I could overlook that they were spying on me, but those concupiscent pigs were satisfying their abusive lust at the expense of Bonita. The guys were enjoying it a lot, and I could even hear them clearly saying Bonita's name.

On the other hand, my brother was present and telling them to stop, and that that was not the purpose. He was asking them to delete the video immediately. I couldn't believe what I was hearing. A part of me was getting more and more enraged. Another part kept me in the seat still, advising me not to make a fuss. I could be misinterpreting what they were saying. But I could not stand the strain, and I got up to leave there before going ballistic. In the hall, I met one of my watchmen, who, puzzled, asked me where I was going so annoyed, for I must have looked quite angry. I replied – taking great effort to restrain my anger – that I hoped that I had not heard what I thought I had. I didn't say anything else and got out of there in a hurry. If they were really spying on me, they would have got the message; if not, what I said did not give many clues either. The incident was left behind. No one said anything to me about it. I ended up calming down, and nothing like it happened again. In any case, the ending of this first stage was close.

Phase Transition

I think that my external behavior in society may not have been very unusual. Bizarre things were going on inside my head, but my deeds were only strange when there was nobody around. Even the psychiatrist who sometimes went with my father on his ghostlike visits into my hallucinatory world used to comment that there was no basis for forcibly admitting me for I seemed to be perfectly capable of making a living. I guess that my criterion would not be too realistic, but, on the other hand, my boss let me continue trying to get my part of the work done. There should have been evidence that I was not going to be able to finish it. Shouldn't there?

I was still unable to deliver anything useful. I repeated again and again that I was nearly there. I kept spending my days and nights trying to compile the code. It was not that I didn't know what I was doing. Sometimes I managed to get a program operating, more or less. But it was only a trifle, just the most basic, and also somewhat defective. I don't know whether I would have been able to finish it or not, but at that rate, it would have taken forever.

Until one day, a Sunday, my boss, already desperate, asked me to go to the office to have a meeting. Only he and his wife were there. He was a friendly man, always sympathetic and optimistic, who never raised his voice. However, even speaking with his usual tranquility, he did it with great harshness. I was under tremendous pressure. I knew he was right, just as I suspected there was nothing I could do about it. They admitted part of the responsibility, they both knew that they should not have let things go so far and should have taken me off the project sooner. They demanded a solution, some kind of commitment.

This was a reality check. I don't think that ever in my life had I felt more anguished than during that short space of time, which seemed everlasting. I was about to cry from helplessness and guilt. I realized the state I was in and that any attempt I would make to remedy it would be futile. I just wanted the pressure to end and disappear. My boss's wife, albeit also pushing, had a more conciliatory tone. I guess they realized that I was about to collapse and ended the meeting. I was finally free to go home, carrying an extra burden of stress on my shoulders. I don't know how my body coped with it all without falling down, but the fact is that it did. However, all this accumulation of stress, fatigue, and intoxication would never have a good ending. It seemed that, inside me, there was something like a civil war: one part of my mind consciously pushing me over the edge and another part unconsciously trying to force me to change my attitude by exploiting my fears.

The next day, while I was waiting for Bonita to come home from work, I heard her talking on the street with her parents. This was the first of only two times she appeared in my delusions, and the only time her parents appeared. It seemed that her role, at least on this occasion, was merely auxiliary. The fact was that it was a successful trigger that made me take action and face circumstances. The conversation was about my impending admission to a psychiatric center. Everything was already prepared, and it was going to be that same evening. They would come for me and take me by force. Her parents were trying to persuade Mi Niña to return to live with them. She was reluctant and refused to do it. Contradictory as it may seem, given my behavior, the idea of separating from her, rather than ending up sectioned, jolted me like an electric shock. It acted as a big shove. The time of keeping watchful and waiting was over. I had to take action.

"I am human, nothing human is alien to me", as Terence said. I know that these kinds of decisions are easily forgotten in light of a new day. When the anguish fades away, one comes back to a state much closer to the usual semi-indifference. The ships have to be burned to avoid escape. I picked up the phone and called my boss. I told him that I had to meet with him urgently the next day. I said that I had to talk to him and everyone in the office. I revealed that I had hallucinations and that I couldn't take it any more. I think he was somehow pleased, not that I was ill, but that there seemed to be a way out of my problem. He has always been a lovely person from whom you could expect all his support.

There was still the issue of my alleged captors. A delusional state of mind does not go away just like that. A belief of this type is still there, even if, at the same time, one is convinced that it is false. My altered mind worked that way: contradictions were not a problem, emotions boiled like a witch's cauldron. In the movie *The Last Crusade*, Indiana Jones has to traverse an abyss over an invisible bridge. Though he knows that the bridge is there, it is not easy for him to dare to take the first step. But he ends up doing it and achieves his goal: the Holy Grail. I decided to go straight to the starting point of those who had to take me to my internment: the office building where Bonita and my father worked. I would explain to her everything that was happening. There would be no such paramedics, no such psychiatrists, no such conspiracy, just fantasy. To cope with giants that are actually windmills, one just has to go and grind wheat.

It was still early, and I had to wait on the street for a while. It was already dark. The main entrance of the building looked very wide and all glazed. Occasionally, people came out. It seemed to me that they were wearing white coats; no doubt they were the psychiatric paramedics. The white coats turned out to be overcoats or raincoats. They wanted nothing from me. They had just ended their workday, passing by my side without paying attention to me. I was living in two worlds at once, but one of them was only virtual. It was eerie, even exciting, to watch the change from one world to another, to feel without flinching the fear and the threat grow until it disappear when the reality manifested. This is an example of the value of having a healthy, skeptical attitude to analyze and face thorny situations. An excess of security in your beliefs can be as problematic as a paralyzing hesitation.

Finally, Mi Niña came out. We met, and I breathed a sigh of relief. I could continue to reduce tension by involving more people in my situation. I gave her a play-by-play account of the whole thing. She knew something was wrong, but she had no idea how much. In any case, the first step towards the solution was taken. I felt released. It is absolutely right that talking and sharing experiences is a perfect escape valve for stressful, overwhelming, and oppressive situations.

The following day, I met with my bosses in the office and told them everything. I did not like that they felt guilty for what had happened or, at least, partly responsible. I think they had just had too much patience. Nothing was their fault in any way, but each one is as he is, and we can't stop people from feeling how they feel. Later, I met with my colleagues, including my brother, and I told them the whole story again, even the hallucinations with them as protagonists. It was like improvised group therapy. Everybody said that they already suspected something was wrong inside my noddle, but nobody had imagined to what extent. Now it was they who were hallucinating. They couldn't believe that I could think they would be capable of doing something like that. They were not angry, just surprised. What was also surprising was that, in that state, I had managed to maintain an almost normal demeanor.

I, of course, had decided to stop taking pills. The project would pass into the hands of my workmates. I would work in the office instead of at home so that I could be supervised not to relapse. The latter was a proposal of mine, as well as quite a naive idea. A new Windows NT version had just appeared. They were setting up a new local network, so I would study all the documentation thoroughly to help them to configure it. Besides, there was a new project for which it was necessary to use a well-known database server. There was no one in the company with knowledge about this system, so I would also have to study it to learn how to operate and use it from our applications. I have always liked learning new things. It was something more calming and relaxing; everything seemed to be back to normal.

Hallucinations and delusions disappeared overnight, almost as if by magic. The mission had been accomplished. I seemed to have learned the lesson. Yet, as in many cases like this, the decision did not remain in effect for long.

Twice: Nemesis

Lust for Life

The unease of the withdrawal from my addiction to methylphenidate was similar to that of quitting tobacco. When I stopped taking it, my body returned to functioning as normal. Then, all the accumulated tiredness came to a head. When one gives foreign substances to an organism, it becomes unbalanced. The body produces certain compounds in excess and lacks others. The outcome of withdrawal is always a feeling of physical discomfort. Little by little, things return to a state of equilibrium, and one gradually feels better. It is just about eating and resting well. The physical stage lasts only a few days or weeks, but the psychological one is not so easy. All the rituals involved in substance abuse, repeated many times a day, every single day, for a long time, constitute a very intense learning process. One becomes an expert in smoking, snorting, injecting, or any other simple and repetitive act of this sort.

Learning means developing and reinforcing synapses and ion channels in neurons. Forgetting is the process of discarding them for lack of use, and it can take years. The rituals of addiction are already implanted in the brain as automatisms. When you have recorded one of these automatisms, it is as though the organism assumes that it is something that you must do almost by obligation. There must be some reason for having done it so many times before. Thus, if one does not do it regularly, the brain reminds it.

It is at this point that desire, appetite, or hunger appear, and then the positive feedback loop of anxiety begins. Anxiety is the product of a sort of struggle between the conscious mind, trying to resist impulses, and the unconscious mind, which continually warns that one is not doing something that must be done, that one has a need that has to be satisfied. Anxiety is the addict's worst enemy – much more than the physical nuisance. Psychological disengagement is a very long stage in which an internal fiend tempts you every few minutes. With anxiety, there are three options: if we make it grow, offering a hard resistance to desire, it reaches a maximum and then fades off. If we fall into the temptation, it suddenly disappears, even before satisfying the compulsive desire, just because we made the decision to do it. The third option, the better one, is to learn not to respond to the demands from the beginning; let them pass by without paying them attention. Doing so requires training. One has to learn how to deviate their attention from such an intense commanding. It is just the natural feeling of need that goes with, for example, hunger or thirst; responding to it is in our nature. Trying to trick the body with a harmless substitute has the effect of reinforcing or sustaining learning. It only makes longer the period during which the addict is most sensitive to relapse.

When doctors prescribe a habit-inducing treatment, they usually do not withdraw it at once. One has to stop it piecemeal. I was taking a lot of tablets daily, so I gave all the stash to Bonita for her to supply them to me in a controlled way. I started taking three pills a day: one in the morning, one in the afternoon, and another one at night. When I would get up to go to work, I had a small packet prepared on the sideboard in the dinette. I worked in the office to be watched, or, at least, to feel that way, so that I wasn't tempted to go shopping. I had a line in the morning, a line after eating, and the latest one when leaving.

I had stopped smoking and drinking alcohol for fear of a build-up of heart attack risk factors. It was when I quit smoking – a vice that I'd had since I was thirteen – that I was able to see how anxiety works. Because I was so absorbed in my work, instead of feeling the desire to smoke, there was a kind of mild physical upset, due to nicotine deprivation. When I finally noticed it, I recalled that I had stopped smoking and then I felt an anxiety rise in me. When I concentrated on work again, it faded out, but it would grow when I went back to focus on nicotine hunger.

My body no longer asked me for methylphenidate, it just asked me to perform the ritual of snorting a line, of whatever it was. I went back to tobacco, which is also a stimulant. But not to cigarettes, not to smoking. I knew about snuff through a friend of mine. He had been promoting it for a while in the clubs to get some money. Snuff is powdered tobacco that is inhaled through the nose. It is usually mixed with something that gives it a minty smell, which, on the one hand, makes it more attractive and, on the other hand, irritates the nostrils a lot. One puts a smidgen on the back of a hand or the tip of a finger and gets it in. It is not illegal and it is sold in some tobacco shops. I do not recommend it to anyone – unless you like to drip a kind of dark mud from your very blocked nostrils. Since tobacco is also addictive, this was only paving the way to falling back into my old habits sooner or later.

However, not everything was uncomfortable and difficult during that rehab span. All of this happened in the early spring. I had spent months locked up at home, sitting in a chair in front of the computer most of the time, not daring even to visit my parents. I had sores on my buttocks and legs, like the sick people who spend all day lying on a bed in the same position. I had set up a local network at home. It was not enough for me to have only one computer. I had four. The name I gave it was 'Hades', the underworld of the ancient Greeks. The abode of the dead. The fact is that, when I freed myself from prison and from my self-imposed chains, one sunny morning Mi Niña and I went to take a walk in Madrid's Botanical Garden.

All that exuberant nature surrounding me everywhere gave me a feeling of freedom that I have never felt since. It was a visceral, animal, untrammeled freedom. I felt like a dog might feel when its master takes it to the country, finally releases it, and it starts to run all over the place as if possessed. I wanted to roll on the grass, touch all the leaves, climb the trees. It was a feeling of ecstasy and I felt a burst of desire to move, run, and jump all over. It was like the first step out of jail after a long sentence. I'm not going to say that it was worth everything that had led up to that moment, but it was a compensation that has left me with an unforgettable memory.

In any case, everything was returning to normal. At work, I was learning new things that would be very useful for my future career. At home, I only used the computer to play video games. I could spend hours playing shooters, going through corridors and rooms, loaded with tons of weapons, ammo, and explosives, sweeping away everyone who crossed my path. The whole thing seemed already over. Would someone risk going through all that again, not knowing if the consequences could be even worse? Aye. One tries to understand and infer the reasons that can lead to that. It is easy to find compelling opposing arguments that seem irrefutable. One only gets a feeling of profound incomprehension until understanding comes from looking in the wrong place. There are no reasons that can be expressed with the logic of words. It is something ineffable, visceral, compulsive. Logic is not the only member of the government of the human mind. Nor is it decided by vote on any occasion. It should be clear for a species on the brink of climate and demographic collapse, but the rationalist tradition has masked it behind a naive idealism. It is not difficult to see it in extreme and amplified cases like mine. But, indeed, the mechanism also works in many less obvious ones, in the daily life of all people, ordinary or not so ordinary, vulgar or excellent.

I Man a de Bush Doctor

I have always had a great interest in everything related to nature. I can recall my first book, and myself eagerly flicking through it, for I had not yet learned to read. It was a biology treatise that belonged to my father's cousin, who was then at the university. She gave it to me to entertain me while she dressed up to go out. I looked, fascinated, at the drawings and photos, wondering what all that stuff could be. My parents would often bring us to the countryside where I used to spend a lot of time looking for insects, lizards, snakes, tadpoles, and frogs. I had a little zoo in my room, with all kinds of small bugs and reptiles in boxes and jars with holes in the lids.

On the beach, I also used to spend long hours on the rocks, looking for specimens. Back then, there was still abundant marine wildlife in the breakwaters. A collection of minerals, from a breakfast cocoa-powder brand, made me fascinated in geology too. I came to have a relatively large collection of rocks and fossils, either purchased or found by myself on excursions to the countryside. Although I was just a primary school child, I enjoyed devouring biology and geology encyclopedias. I used to dream of discovering exotic bugs and rocks that could only be found in remote places. Later, I also became interested in botany. Like almost all children, I grew the typical beans or loquat seeds from time to time and amused myself taking care of them and watching their growth.

In high school, I had my first contact and flirtation with joints. This led me to become interested in other vegetable species: *Cannabis sativa* and *Cannabis indica*, marijuana. Having these plants at home meant self-supply of the forbidden; autonomy, independence from both authorities and drug dealers. To be honest, this drug was never my cup of tea. I don't like the effect it produces when you're not used to it, and you're dopey all day when accustomed to it. I need to be active, so I have never really taken a liking to it. I have always ended up quite quickly quitting it, more annoyed than anything else. However, it is a widely spread and accepted product, so it is all around. In the adolescent stage, you are not a cock if you don't smoke even once in a while. My first hemp plants came from bird food; industrial hemp seeds. The plant is similar to that of marijuana, but only in appearance – it is useless for getting high. I didn't know where to find the real stuff; nobody had it, no matter how many people I asked. Nor was there the vast seed market that exists today.

This quest turned marijuana cultivation into a pending topic, more for the mere fact of having hemp than for consuming it. I had little interest, if any, in smoking it. The idea of selling it didn't even cross my mind. I just wanted to have the plants. Mainly because I wasn't allowed to have them. I am such a rebellious guy. One night, at a party, we met and became friends with a couple. They were quite fond of natural stuff, and they also had marijuana plants. Of course, they had seeds, so I asked them for a few, happy that I could finally have the opportunity to satisfy my whim.

To be honest, despite having a fondness for cultivation, I was not an expert. I knew that one had to water and fertilize the crops but little else. Besides, my apartment was not the most appropriate for this type of plant. It had no balconies, just floor-to-floor windows, with a railing to lean out. Though it was the top floor, it only had a few hours of morning sun. I had to hang the flowerpots from the railing to scrape a few more rays of sunlight, so they couldn't grow big enough. Still, I managed to get some plants to thrive, and I had two or three pots on the window. Even though it was not unusual to see hemp plants on the balconies, I knew that you could get done if you were caught by the police. This used to happen as a result of a neighbor's complaint.

The idea was slowly percolating in my mind. But, in the beginning, it was not a problem. It was like having any other plant. They did not grow very fast, due to the small pots and the lack of sun, so they didn't attract much attention. I also did not overthink that they could be a problem. What worried me was that I didn't know how to take good care of them. By then, I was already using the Internet regularly, with the maddening slow phone modems of the time. In any case, it was quite an improvement. Before the net, one had to invest a great deal of time and work in gathering quality information and documentation on any subject. Moreover, not long before a magazine had appeared specializing in the cultivation of marijuana. I began to study everything related to this subject with great care. While I was at it, I learned a lot about many other plants and fungi with tempting properties. There was always an article or document about them, among those on the cultivation of marijuana.

I learned that the flowers of the female plant were what people smoked. I also learned that one could extract the resin from them from which the hash was made. Until then, I thought that people smoked the leaves; one learns something every day. Anyway, it takes many months until the flowers appear, so, from time to time, I would remove some leaves from the plants and let them dry, just to taste it. It seemed to me that the effect was quite remarkable, probably because I was unused to pot. It was also more acceptable than hashish, which was what I had tried so far. So, my consumption was limited to a sporadic dry-leaf joint. Of course, it was only marijuana, because I still didn't smoke tobacco.

Likewise, this magazine regularly reported on the underhand ways resorted to by the police when they busted folk caught growing the plants. Such cheaters would weigh the entire plant without drying it – branches, leaves and roots included – so they could say that they had caught a bigger stash and, at the same time, charge the poor unfortunate of a more serious crime. Sometimes they weighted the plants with soil and anything else, even with the pots. I don't know whether they were just urban legends or all those stories were true. I guess that it was probably a little bit of both.

The point is that the bunch of potential enemies was increasing as the amount of information available on the subject grew. Not to mention marijuana thieves: abject beings who take advantage of the work of others. One takes care of one's garden and, when the fruits of the hard and patient labor are finally ready, the burglars go and steal everything. Possibly along with some other valuable stuff they find in the house.

A Stumble Is Not a Fall

Meanwhile, at work, everything went on as usual. We used to go every day to a bakery in the neighborhood. They would bake some finger-licking good dinner rolls with onion, chorizo, or bacon. Many times, I went there on my own. No one ever took escorting me so that I would not fall into temptation seriously. It was understandable, for they were not my babysitters. The thing was, that between marijuana and snuff, I wasn't developing an attitude consistent with a healthy and abstinent lifestyle. One day, the temptations that intermittently assault those who are trying to quit an addiction, suggesting recalling the old times and wants, managed to win and tip my will towards the decision to buy a box of tablets once again.

In the first days of abstinence from addiction, when anxiety is most intense, it is easy to relapse to escape from that vicious circle. Anxiety can become unbearable, especially for a weakened person with an erratic will. There is another peak in the probability of relapse after a few months. The body is almost recovered, the abandoned vice has been idealized as something more pleasant than it really was, while the bad memories have been losing intensity. In this phase, the relapse is not due to an irrepressible urge – at least not according to my experience. It comes as a decision like any other decision. The fact of making this choice also produces a pleasant and morbid tingling. Perhaps it is the pleasure of breaking the rules, or in particular, even our own selves.

Be that as it may, the organism rewards itself for making this decision, perhaps for a simple biological mechanism without rational explanation. The point is that one decides and does it as one decides and does whatever else one decides and does. We humans are capable of justifying whatever it is if we insist on doing it. There are many standard excuses, which are already a tradition in this field, to which one can resort without making an effort: 'only once and that's it'; 'this time I already know it, and I will be careful', etc. If they do not sound convincing, it does not cost too much to make up another one. It is an inbuilt ability of our species.

The fact was that I returned to the old ways and it was not only once. The fact was also that I was careful and had control, but only for a while. Among the innumerable occasions where I have given up smoking, only once was I able to uphold the goal of smoking three cigarettes a day when I returned to my addiction. I managed to stay that way for several months, but, in the end, I went back to my usual amount. It is a fight that no one can win, although it seems to me that everyone who experiences a similar situation is convinced otherwise. I trusted my will even when it was under my nose that my decisions wouldn't be fulfilled.

It was on the cards that the story would repeat itself. On this occasion, however, there were missing critical and significant factors: pressure and stress. My daily assignments were quite easy. I worked eight hours a day, doing tasks that were effortless for me. When I went back home, at most I played some video games, watched television, or went out for a walk or to a party at night. I had a regular life; there seemed to be no danger. But every addiction generates stress, even if it is just because of the fear of being caught. Fears, along with and amplified by the excitement of stimulants, fuel paranoia. An additional source of concern was the mere presence of marijuana.

Bonita sometimes talked, from window to window, with the neighbor in the building next door. This neighbor had a young daughter, more or less our age. We used to wonder if the neighbors knew that the plants in the window pots were marijuana and whether that would matter to them. We guessed that the neighbor's daughter knew that it was hemp. One day, her mother commented on how beautiful the plants were, how much they were growing. We took it as a kind of ironic warning. Something like: 'I know what you have planted there.' Immediately, I removed the plant pots from the railing of the window of my workroom and put them on the sill of the window of the living room. The living room was located to the right of my workroom and out of sight of this neighbor's house, whose balcony was to the other side. On the balcony of my workroom, I placed ivy to hamper the view of the pots. Thus began a kind of game of cat and mouse that was going to get worse and worse.

One can wonder, and it is a reasonable question: Why not change the cultivation of marijuana for geraniums, for instance, and stop complications? After all, for me, pot was not exactly a delicacy. Honestly, I have no answer to that question. That's how stubborn I am, I guess. I wasn't going to throw in the towel so soon. The situation was not so bad; I just had to hide the plants well so that the neighbors could not see them. A bit like a gentleman's agreement: do not show them to me, and I will pretend I do not know that you have them. Complicating my life, as I think it is becoming clear, is not something that worries me too much. My common sense is different from that of those who do care. Common sense is the least common of the senses, let's not forget.

In any case, I make a living solving problems, so problems for me are the spice of life. This is perfect on some occasions, although it can become an awful thing on other ones. Of course, the least convenient problem for me was the abuse of stimulants. In the beginning, this consumption was quite moderate; after all, my life at that time was quite calm and varied. However, continued use creates addiction, and addiction demands consumption more and more frequently. To avoid taking so many tablets, I started consuming codeine again. Unlike what happened to me with the d-MPH, I never had to take a lot of codeine. The effect lasted long enough for me to take it only three times a day, and it reduced the compulsion to consume methylphenidate so often.

Drugs work by modifying brain chemistry, but the outcome does not depend only on the amount of substance taken. When the body depletes reserves of certain natural compounds, the effect of drugs changes or even disappears. If you take too many stimulants for too long, they can make you sleepy or have no effect at all. If you are an addict, this usually leads you to consume even more, not to stop doing it. The situation was becoming a medication cocktail without any control. It couldn't end well.

Taxi Driver

In a neighborhood, there are always people talking. People are conversing on the street or chitchatting in the surrounding dwellings, sometimes loudly, sometimes even shouting. An inner courtyard is full of sounds and voices. One can hear some television and radio sets, too. The concern about a possible complaint from a neighbor about the bloody grass made me listen attentively to everything that sounded like a conversation around me. I was obsessed with finding out if anyone mentioned the plants placed in my window.

Most of these voices could not be clearly understood – if one single word was. The process that had led me to hear my first surge of voices was being reproduced almost identically. I tried to listen to other people's conversations, filling in the gaps left by the words that I could not understand, and using my expectations to interpret what I feared to hear. In short, I gradually began to feed paranoia.

A family of taxi drivers lived on the first floor of the building. The father and his two older sons shared the father's car. I suppose that doing that they could work for more days a week. In addition to them, there was the mother and the youngest son, maybe ten years old – I'm not good at estimating people's ages. They were good people and always greeted other neighbors cordially when they crossed with them on the stairs. They seemed to get along together and with others. But they had a trait that was going to give me problems: they continually got into quarrels amongst them. Their home seemed like a battlefield. They were one of these families that, still getting along, bedlam erupted every time they argued about something. And they used to do it quite often, unfortunately.

The balcony of their apartment was just below the window of my living room. It was somewhat wider than the rest of the terraces on the facade and protruded. The hemp pots were right in my living room. The marijuana plants had been growing, and with the plants, the size of the pots had also got bigger. The amount of water necessary for irrigation had consequently increased as well. At first, I watered the plants without any care until, one day, I was horrified to discover a waterfall cascading down on the taxi driver's balcony. That was all we needed! Besides attracting attention and bothering others, it was certainly not the best way to encourage them to turn a blind eye.

When one wants to become convinced of something, it seems that the entire universe conspires to come to one's aid. Not long ago, in the 1980s, there was a rise of citizen insecurity caused by the vast tide of heroin addiction. Also, a few taxi drivers had been robbed recently, even resulting in the death of an unfortunate victim. Surely, drugs and drug addicts were not great favourites of taxi drivers. I began trying to understand what they were saying when I heard the yellings from their continuous arguments ascending from the inner courtyard. But, even when they were yelling, it was not easy to understand what they were saying. Anyhow, since I feared or expected to hear the word 'marijuana', it ended up appearing every now and then, with increasing frequency.

The first thing I had to do was solve the water problem. That was fairly easy: I just had to put the plants inside the flat. I cleared the corner to the right of the window in my workroom, and there I placed the pots. The marijuana had finally disappeared from the sight of the neighbors – one fewer problem. The worst was that the plants needed sunlight to grow properly, and they did not have it in there. Though it is not the best solution, there are special bulbs and fluorescent tubes that provide a substitute to sunlight for indoor plants. In Hortaleza Street, very close to my home, there were quite a few specialized lighting stores, so there I went looking for these kinds of fluorescent lights. Actually, the best option would have been to use sodium bulbs, but the energy bill would go up quite a bit due to their high consumption. I had read that a sudden rise in electricity consumption could be a suspicious sign of illegal crops. The bulbs also produced a lot of heat, and I would have had to set up ventilation systems. There were too many complications. It seemed better to opt for fluorescents; not so efficient, but less consumption. I placed them on the walls around the plants.

The few fluorescent tubes that I could put up did not give enough light though. I would have to put up more, and of the longest ones, or the plants would not grow properly. I saw the solution one day as I passed a rubbish bin: a discarded door, which I, triumphant, immediately picked up and took home. I hung the door horizontally with ropes above the plants, leaning it against the wall, and I put another four of the longest tubes I could find on the door. Now there did seem to be enough light. Problem solved. But the anger of my taxi-driver-neighbor did not seem to disappear along with the plants. Instead, the opposite happened: its intensity increased because he felt mocked, for he could no longer demonstrate my connection to the underworld. When we crossed each other on the stairs, they continued to greet me in a friendly fashion, although I used to feel grim glances and whispers behind my back. They had it in for me, in particular the father. They were after me.

I used to hear their uproar from the kitchen window, which faced the inner courtyard, and I would lean out as much as I could, trying to understand most of what they were saying. These neighbors also used to screech in casual conversation. Albeit I was trying to eavesdrop on them surreptitiously, I felt that they somehow realized this. That increased their anger towards me. No one likes to be spied on, even though he is himself spying on the spy. But they were talking about me all the time, and they were rude. I had to do something. The auditory hallucinations had reappeared, hand in hand with paranoia.

They felt entitled to spy on me, spend all day talking about me, plotting dark revenge. But I was not allowed to listen to them, as they used to tell me. They were so cocky. I discussed my fears with Mi Niña, who was not quite sure whether to believe me or not. I used to advise her to beware of them, just in case. For their part, they were very offended by my suspicion that they were going to do something to her. She had nothing to do with the brawl, they said. At some point in my rage, I made an inopportune comment about his car; to scratch it, to slash its tyres or some such threat that is sometimes made. That, of course, made them mad. I was suggesting outright that I was going to attack their livelihood! I never intended to do anything to their cab, of course. It was just the typical outburst that one vents. Instead, the one who feared for his physical integrity was me: They were many; they were aggressive; I had no chance against them. I also had no evidence with which to report them to the police. They were developing a visceral hatred of me that seemed totally over the top. All I could do was avoid meeting them in the street or on the stairs. This time, my body's response to the toxic aggression was not going to be kind.

On one occasion, I was tempted to call the police to intervene, but, fortunately, I did not. I was at home, on a work meal break. Every day I went back home for a change of air and to have a meal. Thereby I avoided interacting too much with my colleagues, lest they notice something odd about me. I also used to take the opportunity to stop by a pharmacy and buy supplies. As I was leaving to go back to work, I suddenly heard some fierce screams, yelling to me to go down to the street. There, my neighbor was supposedly waiting for me with a baseball bat or something similar to beat me up finally. I froze without daring to leave home. I waited a while to see if he would get tired and go away. But no way; he was still there, shouting and asking me to come down, and that I was going to find out what was what. I could have called the police, but looking out of the window, I couldn't see the lunatic anywhere. Surely that was what he wanted: I would call the police, and then they would think I was nuts. When the officers would arrive, he would no longer be there; when I would bring them up to his home, my neighbor would deny everything, absolutely weirded out. No one is capable of imagining more twisted plans than a paranoid.

If this was the case, it would be just a ruse, so I could safely go down to the street. As I was hesitating about whether to leave home or not, time was passing, and I was getting late for work. I phoned to say I was late for I was having trouble with a neighbor. Then, I still floundered for a while. On the one hand, I had to leave to go back to the office; on the other hand, there was the fear of a potential beating. The taxi driver was nowhere to be seen. I was ruminating the possibility that the whole thing was happening only inside my mind, of course. There were precedents and reasons. But the intensity of the experience significantly reduced confidence in this possibility, although it was by far the most reasonable explanation. Again, the most visceral emotions dominated reason. It is almost impossible to resist what the senses tell us.

The point is that, in part because the neighbor seemed to stop bellowing, and partly because I took courage, I ended up going out. There was nobody there, as expected. Everything seemed peaceful, as usual in those early afternoon hours. I went back to work, suspecting that I would have more encounters like this with the taxi driver and his two older sons, who were much less pugnacious, but who naturally supported their father. Hostilities had been definitively declared.

Daddy, Daddy!

Not everyone in the taxi driver's family had turned on me, though. The mother seemed to like nothing at all about the direction the situation was taking. Her roars were directed at her husband, not at me. She would tell him to drop the matter at once. It was too bizarre an affair. The truth was that I had not really done anything to them; they were overreacting. The remaining family member, the younger son, also begged for the father to calm down and forget about me. "Daddy, Daddy!" I used to hear him say when his father was rabid and seemed like he was going to kill me. And then, a long litany of pleas and exhortations urging him to calm down. "Daddy, Daddy!" he'd say when his father, with his threatening tone, stated that he was going to beat me up. And then the litany repeated again. The poor boy appeared to really suffer from the whole ugly business.

It seemed that, among my hallucinations, there was always someone in the role of advocate. In this case, though, they did not act in my defense but tried to prevent their relatives from getting into trouble. Again, all this stuff came along with a feeling of healthy skepticism. This feeling allowed me to question the reality of this absurd situation. However, in the moments of highest tension, I felt almost complete certainty about the truth of the facts. I suppose that the risk sensation triggered mental alert mechanisms that forced me to feel this way. But, before the situation reached its peak, doubt would be triggered too, which limited anxiety and fear.

When things were quiet – the attacks did not take place continuously, but in waves – I would say to myself that what was happening was not possible, and I tried to persuade myself of it. Indeed, when I was in good spirits, if I met my nemesis on the stairs, I would dare to exchange a few words with him, to observe his reaction. The thing is that he reacted normally, talking to me in a friendly way, like any neighbor, as if nothing strange was going on. After all, he was an ordinary neighbor, and nothing weird was really happening. This was a huge relief to me but it didn't serve as conclusive and definitive proof of anything.

Having recently experienced a situation in which I had heard voices, which were clearly nothing more than a product of my mind, did not seem to tip the balance decisively towards reality. Knowing that if I stopped taking the d-MPH the voices would disappear also had no effect on forcing me to do so. In this case, doubts acted in favor of delirium. If the situation was real, stopping taking the pills would only weaken me. In such circumstances, despair is a much more effective ally than reason, and I was not yet desperate.

On the other hand, this time, I had no problem with my job, and my job depended entirely on logic, which on that side of things was working perfectly. The reality distortion seemed to work selectively. It was applied to specific people and situations; the rest stayed unaltered or altered only to a small extent. All the other neighbors seemed as normal to me as they ever did. When one is addicted to whatever it is, one devises an alternative, absurd as it may be, to the most intelligent and appropriate solution for the problem: stopping the addictive behavior or consumption. One magnifies the suffering that abstinence could entail, which actually, is usually much less than one expects, and minimizes the perception of harm. I will quit it at a better time…

My taxi-driver-neighbor used to check his car quite often, on the street, in front of the building. This was irksome, for it forced me to pass by him whenever I was entering or leaving. The fact that he had a wrench or any other blunt object in his hands was not reassuring. Luckily, his youngest son was usually with him on these occasions. "You'll see," the taxi driver would say for instance, "he is going to find out who I really am!" "Daddy, Daddy! No!" the child always replied, followed by the usual chain of pleas. And the father listened to him, stayed still, and went on with his business. "I just say it to scare him!" he sometimes said. And I would pass by them pretending not to be listening, ignoring them if they ignored me, and greeting them if they greeted me. Keeping my troubles to myself.

Meanwhile, my physical condition was also worsening. I was getting slimmer and weaker again. My job was getting weightier as well. Actually, everything was weighing me down. I could work as usual, but I felt less and less like doing it. The stimulant tablets often caused me unavoidable drowsiness that made me think I was going to fall asleep suddenly. We used to have quite a few work meetings, and many of them were after lunch in the early afternoon. Staying awake was a titanic task. I couldn't use stimulants because the solution was worse than the problem. Still, I would be forced to do it every so often, driven by addiction.

It is incomprehensible why I did not immediately opt for the simplest solution and abandon the vice. Especially considering how little it costs to give up an addiction when you really are willing to do it, compared to how bad it is to hold onto it against all the odds. But we stubbornly persist in painting a very black picture of the process. We can develop a visceral feeling of rejection and a tremendously strong resistance to the idea. Making the decision can take months, years, or a whole life. Over time, I have learned to ignore my expectations. One faces the situation, and we'll see what happens. The reality is out there. Inside our minds, there are only omens.

I was beginning to consider the idea of stopping work altogether for a while, to have a respite. In this way, I could also take the opportunity to stop snorting tablets. If I had no duties, I could be relaxed at home, recovering from my ills. I would have fewer excuses to delay the decision. Quitting addictions is not like removing a tumor. Somehow it feels like one is going to lose something of oneself, a piece of one's personality. Either one rejects that habit entirely, or one hangs on to it with tooth and nail. It is a toxic relationship with oneself.

Conspiracy Nut

My hostile neighbors' flat was not the most suitable for spying on me. They lived on the first floor, I lived on the fourth. From their home, they couldn't see inside mine. But soon, they managed to get more resources. They were not only outnumbering me, they were not only physically stronger and more aggressive than me, but, alas, they also had other relatives close by to ask for help, as is often the case with violent clans.

In the building across the way, also on the first floor, lived another family, made up of quite a few members, and they were related in some way to the taxi driver or his wife, I don't remember which. The fact is that they were soon recruited for the surveillance tasks that my foes could not undertake. It was not the best position, as it was still the first compared to the fourth floor, but at least it was in front of my windows and not below. The black ops of this family were carried out with neither enthusiasm nor belligerency. But even so, they reported to the quarrelsome taxi driver on everything they managed to observe. The taxi driver was very demanding; indeed, it seemed that he was oppressive to them as well, but family is family.

This time, there was no cutting-edge technology, but the traditional system of looking through the slits of blinds and curtains. It was so annoying to draw so much attention from more and more neighbors. They were making a big deal out of it. There were just a few plants. I know it was a drug, but its consumption was already as widespread as that of tobacco. It was something almost entirely accepted by society. It was clear that I was not, and did not intend to be, a pusher. It was the typical quarrel among neighbors that begins with some minor nonsense and can potentially end in a massacre. The most querulous, resentful, and vindictive face of common people. A cliché, a stereotype. My new voices were built using stereotypes. It didn't matter how ridiculous and absurd they became. It was as if I believed that one can expect something terrible from people if no one is watching them. I was creating a fictional world in which anarchy and abuse prevailed. On the other hand, I was also able to observe the real world without finding a trace of people like these. It didn't matter, because I would always end up thinking that they were an exception and that I had had the bad luck to meet them. Occasionally, on the news, one can see some case that allows justification of this.

Several factors were preventing me from making the simple decision to get rid of the plants. On the one hand, it was a matter of pride and dignity. I wasn't going to let them step all over me like that. On the other hand, the plants weren't really the issue anymore; they were a simple excuse. The subject had become a personal matter and it would be pointless to get rid of them. There was also the doubt, the everlasting doubt: what if it turns out that, as it is much more reasonable to suppose, all this is only inside my head? Doubt hinders decision making. If one wants to avoid making a decision, all that one has to do is generate all kinds of uncertainties that prevent one from making it. For us humans, doubting is much more reasonable than being sure, so justifying doubts is straightforward.

The heuristic I used was not based on incorrect logic. In fact, it was entirely consistent if all the premises were considered valid. It was the same logic that allowed me to perform in the real world, just that I was much more open than the average person to accept as possible things that usually seem impossible to us. The real world belongs to the realm of physics rather than to that of logic. Physics is not based on logic. The force of gravity is not logical at all. It is there, and we can feel it, but even Newton found it incredible that action-at-a-distance could exist. He accepted it because his senses and experiences told him to, not because it was logical. If I can be a nut, why can't others be nuts too?

Something happened, to top it off, that added even more characters to the bunch. The building where Mi Niña, Gato, and I lived in was an old one, and old buildings often need renovation from time to time. The time came to renovate it, and it required significant repair: roofs, staircase, plumbing, and facade. A lot of time, a lot of work, and many workers. Workers everywhere and all the time. Scaffolding on the facade and roofs full of people. The thing did not look good.

The workers, of course, had nothing against me, at least in the beginning. The boss was a pretty nice guy. We talked to him a few times because we had the access keys to the roof, and they had to fix the glass skylight that crowned the staircase. The glass roof was broken, and the rainwater poured through the cracks, causing puddles on the wooden stairs, which deteriorated them more and more. My problems with them began with an unfortunate event that, in my feverish and paranoid imagination, earned me their eternal enmity and threw them into the arms of my delusional nemesis: the psycho taxi driver.

One day they told us not to use the bathroom or, if we did, not to flush, for they were going to be fixing the waste pipes. So we were very obedient when we got up in the morning to go to work. Like every day, I returned home at lunchtime. After lunch, just before leaving to go back to work, I felt the need to visit the crapper. Absorbed in my thoughts, it was an unfortunate automatic reaction to flush the toilet when I had finished, already in a hurry because I was a little late. A rush of imprecations, curses, and oaths in Aramaic rose through the inner courtyard to tell me that I had made an unforgivable mistake. All was not lost yet; perhaps I would have time to escape unseen. After all, I was not the only neighbor in the building. So I sneakily left and went back to the office. I didn't cross anyone on the stairs or in the doorway. No one ever mentioned the incident to me, so I can't know for sure whether it actually happened or only existed in my creative psyche.

The malevolent taxi driver was quick to recruit the workers for his cause, speaking against me all the time. I could hear them talking in the courtyard or on the stairs. They were already an army, a horde. Even so, I still stuck to my guns. We can have ingrained in us so deeply vices, habits and customs that we are capable of exposing ourselves to the worst kinds of deaths rather than letting them go. If we were able to channel at will all this power towards higher goals, the human species would only be composed of geniuses.

The only advantage I still had against the Army of Shadows was that all of its troops had a real, palpable human counterpart. I just had to have a casual conversation with any of them to realize that they were ordinary people who apparently had nothing against me, nor seemed to be aware of the battles fought against their avatars in my inner world. It didn't work perfectly, but it did it a little, feeding the doubt that constituted a kind of escape to reality.

Of course, they could be dissembling, not showing their cards, for me to become confident and be off guard. But it didn't seem like it, and that's what mattered. Different trends in the physical or emotional state of the organism can be raised by merely exposing something to the senses. This is what happens with the placebo effect: you take a pill, and you feel better. It doesn't matter whether the thing is actually a piece of candy; improvement even depends on its color or shape. Actual people were my placebo against their avatars: they didn't cure, but they did alleviate the symptoms.

This time, fortunately, no one had the keys to my apartment, not even the landlords, since I had added new locks to the door. The scaffolding had not yet been assembled as the facade was to be at the end of the renovation, so I still had a reasonably safe stronghold against my attackers. Attackers who, for whatever reason, seemed unwilling to carry out their threats. Nor did they appear to be very successful in gathering information that could be used for a possible complaint with the police. At the moment, we were at an impasse.

Follow the Light

One may wonder how someone who is living in a situation like that can appear normal to others, but there is an easy recipe: don't tell anyone. My profession provides a particular advantage in this regard: a software developer can be strange and uncommunicative and still be considered 'normal'. I had no hallucinations or delusions related to the programming of applications and databases, just as I did not have them with Bonita, Gato, or the rest of my neighbors. Nor were the hallucinations with my co-workers or family members back. Part of my world was weird and quirky, but it was mostly still the real world as we all know it. It was like living in a secret adventure: a play within a play. I don't know how I did it, but I carefully selected the actors. My hallucinations were something private, a world to which only I had access. It was seemingly as real as life itself, though incredible and inaccessible to the rest of the mortal world. A parallel dimension.

When I speak of apparent normality in my demeanor, this is not to say that it was the kind of normality to which everyone is used. Normality, in my case, meant being proficient to work, being able to have coherent conversations with others. I was capable of fending for myself. Notwithstanding, my physical aspect was not exactly healthy. I was gaunt and getting thinner; I was always tired. Sometimes I had moments of absence when I listened to the voices at the same time as to Bonita, and I could not pay attention to what she was saying to me. The sleepless working nights were over, but I didn't rest well. Mi Niña, as she was living with me, noticed something odd, though. She knew I was taking d-MPH, but not to what extent. It worried and saddened her. It made her suffer. Sometimes I seemed almost a stranger to her. No, it wasn't the normality that healthy people are used to, just the absence of loss of contact with reality, of total alienation.

The days passed under that ever menacing sword of Damocles that was my obdurate taxi-driver neighbor. I was subjected to the surveillance of his relatives from the opposite building. In the same way, the gang of workers stalked me in mine. The threats were never carried out, and the espionage never seemed to lead to anything. However, all this stuff had the effect of keeping me in a constant state of tension, alert to every detail. One afternoon, when I came back home from work, I observed from the street the window of my workroom, where the marijuana plants were, to get an idea of the perspective that my neighbor's family members had on it. It was the time of year where it was getting dark at that hour. The window was emitting a suspicious bluish light, sort of making my room look like a spaceship. It certainly wasn't a normal light for a typical home. I had never noticed it before. My hideout was not perfect. During the day, the shine was masked by the clarity of the environment. However, at nightfall, it became a beacon that could attract the attention of the entire neighborhood (and probably anyone else who passed by on the street). I had to solve it somehow, since turning off the fluorescent lights at lunchtime would deprive the plants of too many hours of light. I was somewhat obsessed with their care. I even provided them with an extra oxygen dose by inserting containers with hydrogen peroxide amid the pots. I also gave them an additional supply of carbon dioxide through a system of pipes that went through the door that held the fluorescent lights over them. I bought the best fertilizers… I ensured they didn't lack anything.

The solution to the light problem serendipitously appeared one evening when leaving home to go and buy something. I was used to inspecting every rubbish bin that I could find on my way, just in case I saw anything useful. What I found on that occasion was a mechanical timer, something like a home electricity meter, which allowed me to program the hours where the lights would be on. It was in perfect condition, and I promptly installed it to control the on and off of the fluorescents. I was obsessed with taking care of all the details so as not to make any mistakes. This, in turn, deepened my mistrust and my suspicions towards all my neighbors—whether they were known or unknown. It was just one more vicious circle.

Besides the thorough and obsessive care of my plants, another of my habits that had become compulsive was the collection of computers and other old electronic devices that I had found in the rubbish. Occasionally, I would find, pick up, and take home one of them, obsolete, though still in good condition. If the finding occurred on the way to my workplace, I used to bring the junk to the office. At the end of the day, I would go back home on the subway carrying the appliance. I have never had a car nor even a driving license (I think luckily for everybody). At home, I used to disassemble them with the idea of reusing their parts in some supposed future invention. Hard drives, video and network cards... all had some value. It was like Dr Frankenstein's lab, but with computers and electronics instead of monsters. All ended up stored in the interior room of the apartment – the closet room – which soon became my private junkyard. It was a bit like Diogenes syndrome. Those affected by this disorder collect everything they find on the street and store tons of rubbish in their homes.

In my case, the collection was selective but also obsessive. I would use what I collected, sometimes only to disassemble and manipulate it. I had my limits in terms of the space that the junk could take up. Otherwise, Mi Niña would put the limits. I threw away everything that I had no choice but to throw. Finding space to store everything was another of the activities to which I dedicated my free time. I reorganized all this stuff over and over again, to stock as many things as I could in the least possible space. It was all free, so the limit was set by the available space. It was another vice, a new mania.

Because of this mania, I added another fifth computer to my underused network. I couldn't handle all five computers at the same time and I had to move from PC to PC. I used to install and uninstall programs and little else, constantly reorganizing everything. But I ended up getting bored and went back to playing video games, as usual. My main goals when I started to set up the net were learning how to do it and being able to play with other people, shooting and chasing one another. But I didn't know anyone interested in it. Bonita doesn't like games, and much less the violent ones. My workmates did like them, but they seldom visited us. Our relationship, although a good one, was not far beyond the job. I even mentioned it to my enemies, Taxi Driver & Sons. I used to talk to them from places in my home where I could hear and understand them, thinking that they could do the same with me. These places were near the windows overlooking the street or the inner courtyard. Once, hearing their usual threats, I proposed that they should come upstairs to play a game to make peace. The sons were more or less up for it, the youngest one liked the idea, but the father, my arch enemy, sent me to hell with profound contempt. "This is a serious dispute," he said, "not a child's fight." It was not going to be solved by playing.

Fate luckily stood in the way of their plans, which would not culminate successfully this time. One happy day, I saw my oppressive neighbors packing their belongings and loading them in the car. They were moving. I felt immense relief. It was the perfect solution, and without any need for intervention, either from me or anyone else. Only one of the older sons remained in the house, but he abandoned the fight; it was not his war. He never played a role in my delusions and hallucinations again. His relatives remained on the opposite floor, and so did the workers in my building, but they posed no threat once their leader disappeared; chances were they would forget about the matter, too.

I never knew what the name of the taxi driver was, or, if I ever knew it, I have forgotten even that. Nor do I remember the name of his sons or his wife. On their side, they never came to know the ignominious role they had played. But the story was not finished. There was still marijuana, d-MPH, and, as I would discover later, almost any instrument that could be assigned some suspicious role, ridiculous as it was. I could still build a more oppressive, more threatening, and broader scenario. The game was not over.

Thrice: Be Fruitful and Multiply, and Fill the Mind and Subdue It

Peace after the Storm

The retreat of Taxi Driver, my major menace, was a relief, but not a solution. The problem was still there, inside me. My paranoia was still active, and it was feeding and growing. I used to scan the neighboring buildings searching for suspicious dwellers, trying to catch conversations that would give them away. Some flats appeared to be uninhabited. In other ones, someone appeared from time to time on the balconies. I was primarily concerned with those windows with clear views over the inside of my home. The attic that was just in front of my apartment worried me in particular. It was not one of those penthouses that had large terraces and windows, but it was a loft with medium-sized skylights in the roof. To see my home from there, one had to stick one's head out. Or have a periscope, or a camera…

I also observed with suspicion the rooftops and the small windows that are usually high up in the old buildings' facades. The attic in front of my flat was clearly unoccupied but, from time to time, potential tenants visited it. Sometimes I could hear voices that seemed to comment on the state of the apartment, its advantages and disadvantages. Not all the talking I heard was about me. That meant that I could discriminate. I wasn't paranoid. I knew how to differentiate between one conversation subject and another.

New neighbors could signify further trouble. I speculated as to the kind of people they could be. The neighborhood was peaceful, with many unoccupied apartments in front of mine. I didn't want to have any more worries. On one of these visits, I saw emerge, through one of the attic skylights, the heads of a series of young guys and girls. Surely they were checking the views. I remember that I imagined that they could be a group of cadets from the Guardia Civil (Civil Guard), a Spanish militarized law enforcement agency. I wasn't really serious, more like half-joking with myself. That would be quite a good booster for paranoia!

The Civil Guard, in a big city like Madrid, was perhaps not the security corps that I had most to fear from. The National Police would have been a more plausible choice. I think the idea came to my mind because of the news I read now and then about marijuana seizures. They appeared regularly in the specialized magazine that I read religiously. The police were not interested in arresting anyone with one or two small plants on their balcony. They would be overwhelmed. What they were looking for were large plantations devoted to drug trafficking. As these plantations were usually located in the countryside, it was usual for them to be dismantled by the Civil Guard, which is the corps that has jurisdiction in rural areas.

The incident with Taxi Driver had had completely drained me and made me decide to stop working for a while and try and quit the drugs again. I thought about redirecting my career, too. So I spoke to my bosses anew to inform them of my decision, and I stayed at home all day, most of the time alone, this time with no work responsibilities.

I used to spend a long time playing with my favorite video games and watching cartoons on TV channels for children. Cartoons have fascinated me since I was a little child, and so they have continued doing over time. The more brutal the stories, the better: explosions, falling, crushing, slashing… As a child, I also loved comics. I used to devour all kinds of comics: fun, far-fetched, and even, of course, violent. The smacks and explosions followed one another, blended with the craziest situations and dialogues. It was inspiring. The fantasy, the absurd and the surreal hypnotized me. In literature, science fiction is my favorite genre. In painting, it is surrealism.

I also felt compelled to devise and draw my own characters. The realistic style was not my thing; too difficult. My realistic drawings totally sucked, so I drew comic-book characters, with big noses, huge mouths and eyes, and all those kinds of things. Everyone used to be amazed that I managed to give them great expressiveness. I drew a complete collection of comics, with many characters, which were also quite violent. It seems that, back then, I had a lot of aggressiveness inside me. I don't like violence in the real world at all; in fact, I hate it. I've always shied away from fighting. But in fantasy, when it's not meant to be realistic, I find it fun and exciting. I don't think it does any harm. It gives me the feeling that it allows us to channel aggressiveness harmlessly, like when hitting a punching bag. My brother and I played endless wars with our plastic soldiers between good and evil, with many characters of our invention. Each war could last for months. We talked to each other through these invented characters; we hardly communicated in any other way.

In high school, I also spent more time drawing than taking notes. I still keep dozens of those drawings, most of them quite surreal. In those pictures appear many characters of my invention, each more absurd than the previous. Many of them also contain violent scenes. There was a time when I even considered studying for a fine arts degree. Nowadays, I still often mentally create crazy new characters. Anyone who frequently appears on television or any advertisement inspires me. I use these made-up characters to illustrate my continual speculations on all kinds of subjects. At the same time as I am turning over a certain issue, I am staging in my mind examples of it in ad hoc situations. Thinking that way is more fun and motivating.

Further, I have had other influences that are much more negative and problematic. I remember that, from a very young age, when watching movies, I used to like the bad guys better than the good ones, except for the rule-breakers, like Dirty Harry. The excessively evil characters, such as the murderers and rapists, always produced in me an intense rejection, though. This fueled in me a romantic vision that, in my adolescence and early youth, led me to explore underground environments, almost criminal. I got into trouble, although much less than one might guess. I was afraid of this kind of people, but I felt safer next to them than in front of them. I never fell into the abyss, but I got very close. I never hurt or attacked anyone. The bonds with my family, to whom I often gave grief, kept me within limits that I did not feel capable of crossing. I did not belong to that world. It was more like a tourist trip: it was adventure tourism. I also got used to dealing with dangerous people and seeing the police from the other side.

Returning to the story, my need for activity soon began to make me feel quite remorseful for wasting time so unproductively. I had to do something constructive, and I didn't want it to be something that required the use of a computer. I've always liked making things. My first job was at a company devoted to manufacturing electronic and mechanical devices for special education. My main task was to design and develop video games. However, in periods when I had less work, they used to assign me to the workshop to help prepare product pieces or assemble and test electronic component boards. This provided me with a lot of training in the use of mechanic tools and practical knowledge of electronics, which complemented those from college.

Therefore, I decided to resume these skills, this time as a hobby, to continue learning. Something fundamental when one's trying to stop drugs is to have an exciting activity to spend the time doing and, above all, to divert attention from temptations. Thus, I invested some money to buy components, tools, and some other bits and pieces, and I got all hands on deck. I also bought some chemicals and vessels to make the printed circuit boards, something that was going to bring me some additional bother.

Because of my particular technological version of Diogenes syndrome, the systematic hoarding of all kinds of devices that could contain electronic circuits was accentuated: radios, TV sets, video players... I used to bring everything home to disassemble and take out components. It was a free source of material, and soon my home was full of containers with resistors, diodes, transistors, capacitors, as well as a variety of buttons, connectors, and cables. They are tiny objects, some minuscule, so I could store thousands of them in very little space. Then I had to classify them. I had jars, boxes, and compartmentalized cases aplenty. But I couldn't have them all in a jumble. Finding something would take hours. This became a new chaotic and obsessive activity: each new classification criterion would be later improved and expanded. I reclassified everything over and over again. I had to redistribute the mess of junk to make room for the new acquisitions.

Order and disorder alternated since, for each new project, I had to select all those elements that could be useful to me. Soon, another new idea would come, leading me to drop the old one. I used to pile the items selected for the abandoned projects somewhere, waiting for the time to return all the stuff to its place. This time, however, there was no external pressure. I did this as a hobby and nobody expected any results. I could take my time with the utmost tranquillity. But I kept going in circles. I spent many hours locked in the inner room, selecting and rearranging everything, snorting another methylphenidate tablet every now and then.

Mus

One day, the feline branch of our family expanded with the addition of a new member. Bonita brought home a small grey tabby kitten. He had a white belly and part of his paws were white, as if wearing socks. His face was all eyes, eyes wide open, inquisitive and pleading eyes, outlined with thin black stripes. On his little orange nose there was a rosy stain that gave him a mischievous air. He was tiny, newly weaned. He had appeared one day in the window display of the pet store where we bought food for Gato. He came from another customer's litter who gave them up for adoption. Mi Niña fell in love on the spot when she saw him in the shop window, begging her with his eyes to adopt him. Something similar had happened with Gato. One day I saw him as I was going to work in the morning, and he looked me straight in the eye. Gato's was not a pleading stare but deeply friendly and intelligent. I had an irresistible desire to take him home right away, but there was some guy around, and I thought the cat was his, so I didn't. It didn't matter, because when I got back home, the cat was already there. Bonita had come across him too, and she couldn't help but pick him up. Cats choose you as much as you choose them.

We called our new friend 'Mus', because a workmate of Mi Niña told us that it means 'cat' in Guinea. Gato never liked the idea too much. He had been dethroned from his position as lord of the manor, and it took some time for him to forgive Bonita. He would turn his back on her when she spoke to him, with the disdain and aristocratic indifference that only cats know how to convey. Mus tried insistently to approach Gato, who rejected him by emitting loud hisses and backing away from him with great irritation. They never became friends entirely, at least on the part of Gato, who seemed to be martyred by the constant hugs and persistent attempts to play from his younger and restless partner. Mus also used to pounce on Gato's bowl like a piranha when we fed them both. Gato stared at us as if to say: "Well, aren't you going to do anything?" We had to separate them at mealtimes.

Since I was at home all day, I became his official caregiver. Being such a small cat, he constantly demanded care. And he was always hungry. A starving kitten is like a machine that emits continuous and sharp meows that pierce the eardrums without mercy. Miii, miii, miii...! Kittens do not ask for food, they impetrate it. There is no alternative but to feed them *ipso facto*. No door can mitigate enough that kind of sharp needle that sticks in one's nerves. As he was so small, it didn't seem suitable to give him cat food, so I fed him baby food. I added it to the d-MPH tablets in my regular visits to pharmacies. Mus devoured it eagerly, at a dizzying pace. That was a bit expensive, but the pussycat induced in me a deep maternal feeling, so I had no choice. My emotions were quite altered.

The main problem with cats and their food is that they are soon sick of even the most delicious delicacies. The food they gobble up today with intense waves of pleasure, can be rejected tomorrow as if it were the most disgusting slop. This meant that I could not store a large batch of food, for I could end up having to throw it away. Often I had to find and buy new flavors with which to surprise my whimsical and spoiled kitty. This meant the added problem of leaving the fragile creature alone and helpless at home. On leaving, I used to feel like a mother abandoning her baby. I always tried to get back as soon as possible. I was developing a strong emotional bond with Mus, and the same seemed to be happening to Mus with me.

At night, the little mister also had to be taken care of. Bonita refused to let him sleep in our bed. We could accidentally crush him. He could also prevent us from sleeping, becoming a torture tool. He used to elicit Gato's anger with the corresponding nightly fuss. Any slight movement under the covers became a prey to be captured with his sharp-like-a-razor claws and teeth. Our fingers and toes became coveted trophies for the unruly Mus. We decided that he should sleep locked up in the living room. But to intend something it is not to get it. Locking the kitten in the living room triggered an inexhaustible siren of meows that made it impossible for us to sleep – and, we suspected, the rest of the neighborhood as well. First, we had to get the cat to sleep, as is done with human babies. To Mus, the most relevant part of a person was the face. This was the only thing that mattered to him. It wasn't sufficient to pick him up and cradle him. He had to see my face. I had to keep my eyes on his big eyes until he fell peacefully asleep. So, when Bonita went to bed, I still had to wait a while to do the same, with the cat curled up in my lap, reassuring him with my gaze like a devoted mother. More reinforcement for the emotional bond. When, finally, Mus felt into Morpheus' sweet arms, I laid him gently on the living room floor, on a makeshift crib made with a folded towel, and there he stayed, sleeping peacefully until the next morning.

In addition to eating and sleeping, Mus used to spend the day playing. All the small objects that came within his reach would end up under some piece of furniture. In my workroom, I had replaced the door with wooden beaded curtains, to have more free space on the walls. Mus used to run through the curtains hunting one end, stretching it as far as possible. And the strings broke, and the beads scattered onto the floor. He never stopped making mischief. He was a continuous bustle. Mus also used to climb the thin railing of the windows that faced the street, and balance precariously before our terrified eyes. We had to cover the fence with wire mesh to prevent him from falling down when the windows were open. We ended up placing wire mesh to completely cover the windows, which gave them a somewhat weird appearance and prevented us from leaning out.

During this time of downtime and quietness, with the added responsibility of caring for my new adoptive child, I gradually reduced my tablet intake and began to recover and look better. I had come to resemble a kind of walking skeleton. I used to draw people's attention on the street, and I sometimes heard comments about how thin I was while waiting for my turn in shops or when travelling on the subway. Or maybe they were just voices coming from my own mind, auditory hallucinations; it was already hard to discriminate between them. Even so, it would not have been surprising in either case. I must have a very resistant body – other people in the same situation would have died.

I believe that we are a species of enormous resistance. Mithridates VI was a famous king of the ancient kingdom of Pontus, located more or less in what is now Anatolia. He was a bitter enemy of Rome, against which he fought successfully for quite some time. Legend has it that Mithridates feared, above all else, being poisoned, a fairly common way of ending the kings in those times and one that had been used against his own father in the celebration of a banquet. To develop resistance to poisons, Mithridates took all kinds of toxins in increasingly high doses. Having been defeated by General Pompey, he attempted to commit suicide with poison to avoid capture, but there was no way. He was fully immunized. He had to be run through by one of his officers with his sword. I think my body had also adapted to consuming large amounts of toxins, though they were consuming me little by little.

I hope that no one takes this as an invitation to downplay excesses. Not everyone is so resistant. Many people die the first time they even try a drug. I simply marvel at the resistance that our bodies show to deterioration, that is, the enormous effectiveness of the defense, adaptation, and self-organization mechanisms that are capable of developing beings as simple as the cells that make up our body.

Quousque Tandem Abutere, Mr Tantrum, Patienta Nostra?

Though he was gone forever, the sinister taxi driver had sowed his poison throughout the neighborhood. I could hear a multitude of distant voices. Voices coming from the buildings opposite, on the right, on the left, from those at the rear. They came from everywhere. I couldn't locate them in any specific place. Usually, they spoke in a normal tone, or even softly, as if they wanted to prevent me from understanding what they were saying. Sometimes, I would hear a sudden shout from one of them, and it was not rare for me to discover that it was only a dog barking. Other times, I would end up realizing that it was no more than a television or radio set. But something was evident: a new conspiracy was being concocted in the neighborhood.

The voices did not talk to me, they spoke about me. They seemed to be conversations among relatives or neighbors, in which they tried to decide if I was an ordinary person or a dangerous criminal. There were boys, but never girls. There were a few women, wives and grannies, who were always trying to lighten the mood and calm things down. They seemed wiser and more like peacemakers than the men, but their opinions didn't seem to have much weight. The men mostly seemed to be old or middle-aged. They were the ones who called the shots. In downtown neighborhoods, they are plenty of old people. I suppose my voices were formed following the statistical principle of maximum likelihood. The older ones talked throughout the day, the rest, only at certain times, as if they were out at work or at school. They were all real gossipmongers.

Among the elderly, one whom I nicknamed 'Don Berrinche' (Mr Tantrum) stood out. I was inspired by a character from a comic of my childhood. He was a really grumpy grandpa. He was angry and complained all day. He seemed to be one of the leaders, also, if only by his insistence.

To them, I was suspicious because I was always at home. I didn't seem to be working, and I certainly wasn't then, but I had money. Moreover, I had a marijuana plantation. I was sniffing lines of who-knows-what substance. I had to be a drug dealer or something like that. However, the ghostly neighbors also had their doubts. The voices were not yet decided on whether I was a criminal or not. I didn't seem very dangerous, I spent most of the day alone at home, without receiving visitors, sitting in front of the computer, with my kitten, Mus, on a cushion on the chair beside me – we were inseparable. Not to mention the hours I spent messing around with soldering irons, tweezers, pliers, electronic devices, boards, components, and cables, making unidentifiable gadgets. So much snooping everywhere was getting annoying. This was already going too far. I wasn't causing anyone any harm, I wasn't a nuisance. It was all very stereotyped: old people with little to do and a lot of mistrust towards the youth; ladies who don't like trouble, and bullies who look over their shoulders at the weak ones. They all seemed ordinary people, people from the neighborhood who did not want strange guys around.

When I went outside, I would feel that they were watching me hidden inside their dens, trying to find out where I was going and what I was going to do, whispering behind me like parrots, until I was out of sight. When I went back home, the muffled babbling would begin anew even before I could reach the doorway. This created a highly oppressive environment. Although they were hiding, they didn't seem to mind me noticing. They considered themselves totally entitled to do whatever they were doing, as they saw me as a threat, as though I had been arbitrarily excluded from society, as though I was nothing more than human waste, a derelict. A feeling of deep contempt to my ignominious and abusive vigilantes began to grow inside me. I didn't know how to resort to the protection of the law. I didn't even know against whom I was complaining, or where he was. Neither had I any proof to do so. It was the feeling of powerlessness had by those who know they are victims of abuse, and also who know that the abuser will go unpunished.

But I was not going to give up, overcome by the weight of helplessness and humiliation. I felt anger inside me because of the situation, but at the same time, I harbored a strong feeling of firmness and determination to face the invaders. I didn't know how, but somehow I was going to get evidence to bring that infamous gang of self-righteous hypocrites to justice. I wasn't going to allow them to play with me, or rather, they were going to stop playing. Of course, sometimes, they managed to get on my nerves, and I was struck by aggressive feelings of revenge. I was tempted to leave the laws aside and take justice into my own hands. But something inside me knew that this was not the way. It was not rational. It was like a visceral warning that this could not be done in any way, that it would be a fatal flub, the final error. I felt that the voices were trying to provoke me on purpose so that I would react with violence. They wanted me to end up committing a crime that they could use to lock me up. I wasn't going to be so stupid as to snap at the bait and fall into their coarse trap.

It is possible to capture a voice. Indeed, it is easily possible: just record it, using, for instance, a tape recorder. If one can hear a sound, the microphone will register it as well. Although that wasn't going to tell me who the voice belonged to or where the speaker was, it would at least be irrefutable evidence of its existence. I used to urge Mi Niña to try and listen out for the same sounds I could hear, intending to make her witness to the reality of my experience. I needed to have an ally, someone with whom I could collaborate to resolve the conflict, someone who could attest to my sanity. It was not easy to do anything if I had to hide from the people around me. Bonita was puzzled. She did not believe in the alleged neighborhood plot, even though I tried to explain it to her in the mildest way I could find to make it credible. "Listen," I used to say when the two of us heard people chatting on the street. "Now they are saying this or that!" But she was always uncertain and it was almost impossible to understand more than a few isolated words.

She ended up believing that I was actually hearing something. She did not have the problem of drug addiction, but, at last, she wasn't sure she hadn't heard the same things as me. It is not necessary to be deranged to misinterpret distant conversations if one strives to unravel them. It was as though she believed me, but only half, only partially, which to her was just one more reason for concern. Nevertheless, it allowed me to carry out absurd actions, such as putting a cassette recorder in the window to try and obtain a recording that demonstrated the plot against me. The bad news was that my foes, one way or another, saw me doing it, even though I could not see them at all. They were hidden in their holes. I didn't know where to look, but they did. To have the blinds down was not a solution either. Mi Niña soundly refused. Actually, when I was alone and I tried it, they managed to watch me through any slit in the blinds, possibly using binoculars or something like that, perhaps even a telescope. I thought about exchanging the window panes with one-way mirrors. We could see through from inside, but they would be mirrors from outside. Bonita refused again; she enjoyed the natural light of day. The idea seemed crazy to her (and so it was).

When I started recording, the problem was that the voices immediately went silent. Perhaps the solution would have been to have a device recording all day, but a cassette tape only had the capacity for as much as forty-five minutes, then one had to turn it over. It was impractical. So I used to try and catch them by surprise. On one occasion, I crawled, like an Indian in a Western movie, from the interior of the flat to the living room window, so that they would not see me from outside. There they were, somewhere undefined, with their endless gossip. I started recording, but they soon realized, and then there was an uproar. "He's spying on us!" Mr Tantrum shouted with anger. Seemingly, only they had the right to spy on others. It didn't matter. Now I'd got them. I had caught them by surprise. "Shout, shout, so I'll hear you better!"

Unfortunately, the result was not what I was expecting. When listening back to the tape, the voices did not appear anywhere. The truth is that, in the background, there was a muttering that could have been the chatter of voices, but faraway and completely unintelligible. Again my ear's hyper-specialisation. I could understand what the voices were saying because I had educated my hearing and forced it to do so over and over again. However, a regular microphone did not have sufficient sensitivity. It did not record all frequencies, and, therefore, I could not recognize what the voices were saying on a recording. I would have to think about something more sophisticated if I wanted to get evidence of the crime.

Counter-Strike

I thought I had found the solution to the technical problem of recording the voices in an article from one of my old electronics magazines. It explained how to build a highly sensitive directional microphone – it's similar to a gun, but with a mike instead of a barrel. The mic is made in such a way that it mostly picks up the sound waves it receives from in front of it. A kind of parabolic antenna is added to the device to concentrate the sound waves over the microphone. If we add a good amp to it, we have the perfect gadget for any self-respecting spy or private detective.

Having a home full of junk has many advantages in these cases. You just have to rummage a bit to find the necessary parts for almost any assembly. As a start, I had a good microphone that my bosses had given me a few years ago in the first company I had worked in, dedicated to electronics. I lacked the parabolic antenna, but a visit to the nearest Chinese bazaar provided me with a large tin lid. I made a radial cut to give it the required curvature. I put an old telescopic antenna in the center of the cover. This way, I could adjust the position of the mic inside the parabola. With a broomstick and the wheeled foot of an office chair, the mechanical part was complete. The whole thing was too big to hold in my hand like a gun – it had to be a device with the highest possible sensitivity so that it could trap even the sound of a pin drop.

The mounting of the electronic circuit board for the amplifier was another story. As usually happens with the assemblies that appear in electronic magazines, there was no way of actually putting it in operation. I was able to make the printed circuit board. I found all the electronic components indicated in the magazine – something that is usually not easy. I finally tested the result over and over again, but no sound at all came out of the headphones. The whole process was followed closely by the voices, with their corresponding comments. They wondered, a bit nonplussed, what the heck I was doing.

My ever-present and unwanted audience also saw me messing around with the chemicals and lab glassware that I was using to make the printed circuit board. They soon discovered a new crime to blame me for: I had a drug laboratory. "He has a laboratory!" Mr Tantrum would exclaim over and over again, as an excuse for his actions. It was no use assuring them that it was as harmless as kitchenware. A drug-making laboratory is something much more sophisticated than a few small glass vessels. One needs chemicals which are very difficult to purchase. Either they were absolutely moronic, or they wanted to tease me.

The thing was not working, and the voices sneered at me and my invention, so I had to discard the sodding amp and settle for a vulgar cassette player to complete the artifact. I connected the microphone to the audio input and the headphones to the output. Finally, I managed to hear what the mic picked up, so I got down to work to start the hunt. The truth is that the gadget seemed to work like a charm. I systematically searched the neighboring buildings by sweeping them with the mic. I could listen to sounds coming from other dwellings that I thought I could only hear thanks to the device. Someone washing dishes, some inconsequential conversations, drawers and doors opening and closing… The usual domestic noises, but hugely amplified.

However, I could not locate the source of the voices. I could hear them as usual, but not through the microphone. For a moment, I thought that failure could become a success, for it would prove to me that the voices were not actual people, that they came from inside my head, since they could not be amplified. But it was not the case. My mind refused to consider that as evidence of anything, even though I never heard any of them with the headphones. The voices came from several different places. Certainly it seemed that they only spoke when the mic wasn't aimed at them. Therefore, I disassembled the device and put its components in the mound of junk. Perhaps I would use its parts later for some other assembly.

For their part, the voices began to get very full of themselves, given my futile attempts against them. As they were getting louder, they were also becoming more defined, with more recognizable characters. Their distinctive personalities began to be drawn out, and I could differentiate between them. They became more belligerent, although they still seemed to waver between considering me guilty or innocent. They wouldn't stop commenting on or asking one another questions about me: "He has a marijuana plantation!", "He has a drug laboratory!", "No, man, he is just a bohemian.", "It's not a drug laboratory, it's just to make circuit boards". I particularly noticed the use of the word 'bohemian' to describe me. They used terms and expressions that I wouldn't. They seemed to be other people. They had a very well-defined criterion for being or not being a criminal: work. If I had a job, I was not a criminal, if not, I had to be one, or I would not have money. As stereotypical as everything else about them.

I decided to try my luck doing something that would scare them into stopping bothering me once and for all. A weapon is always threatening enough, so I built a crossbow using two spearguns that I had rescued from – where else? – a rubbish bin. I handled the pieces on the living room floor as though I were an expert gunsmith. I even bought a laser pointer to align the crossbow gunsights. I never had the slightest intention of using it, of course, it was just skullduggery, pure appearance. Needless to say that it didn't have the expected outcome. In fact, it was even counterproductive. To the voices, the ruse did not seem to inspire any fear at all, but they didn't take it well. They were the neighborhood watchmen, the community vigilantes. That made them quite angry. Even though I disassembled the device and returned the parts to the scrap heap, they weren't satisfied. Finally, I had to throw the harpoons away, in what I think was the only concession I ever made to 'them'.

On another occasion, I decided to take a chance with an old pellet gun that I had kept as a childhood keepsake. The carbine was in the closet room, disassembled like all the other items. One of the pieces was a scope sight; nothing spectacular, by the way. It was something akin to a real telescopic sight, but smaller. Sometimes, when I was alone at home, I would turn off all the lights at dusk to see if they could see me then. And yes, they could. Taking advantage of the gloom, I put the gunsight on the living room table, to check if they were impressed. "He has a telescopic sight!" cried Mr Tantrum in alarm. It was not a good idea. This became another justification for his actions: "He has a marijuana plantation!"; "He has a laboratory!"; "He has a telescopic sight!".

As a matter of fact, they seemed like a bunch of imbeciles. Absolutely idiotic. And, worst of all: if it was I who had created them, then I was the most idiotic of them all. I explained to them that I had only tried to trick them, that I had nothing but a disassembled and probably already useless BB gun. But they continued with their mantra and their harassment. Usually, it seemed like they were very, very serious. Sometimes, they said they were just kidding me. On those occasions, there was always someone of them who denied it: "That's not true! He is going to find out what's what". There was no way to ascertain what they wanted. If it had not been for the obstinate siege, for the continuous and persistent meddling, I wouldn't have taken the matter so seriously.

The way of communicating with the voices was somewhat strange and singular. Somehow, they could see me, so the most straightforward system was to start doing something that would transmit a message to them, as in the case of the crossbow or the telescopic sight. I could hear and understand what they were saying. They could realize that by my reactions. Therefore, they could speak to me directly if they chose to. But most often, they would do it indirectly, talking to each other about what they wanted to convey to me. Apparently, they were also able to hear even my slightest whispers, a mystery that I solved with the specious argument that they knew how to lip-read. They were still simply neighbors, ordinary people, though, of course, they were not normal, or perhaps that was the way ordinary people behaved when nobody was watching them. Old ladies, retirees, the average man in the street... they didn't seem to me to be the kind of people who would use sophisticated technologies. But I was beginning to suspect that there was a video camera somewhere, hidden in the recesses of some roof.

I still had contact with my former co-workers. Occasionally, I dropped by the office to chat with them, as they were also my friends. While I wasn't sure whether I wanted to continue to devote my life to coding, my bosses still wanted to count on me for the future, when I was recovered. At the end of the first month, I was surprised to see that I had been paid as usual, although I was not working. I thought it must be a mistake and I went to the office to tell them and return the money. It was not a mistake, they intended to pay me until my recovery. In part, they felt responsible for my condition. I felt terrible and tried to convince them that they were not responsible at all, and that I didn't want to be paid if I hadn't earned it, but they were having none of it. And they continued to pay me the following month, and the one after. I had to start thinking about looking for another job to earn a salary and get them to stop giving me money, at least until I was clear on whether I wanted to continue with my usual profession, in which case, of course, I felt compelled to return to work for them.

At that time, too, an event happened that meant a radical change in the tense situation I was experiencing. It happened about the time Bonita used to come home from work. Somehow, our cats realized that she was home even before she came through the door, perhaps on hearing her take out the keys. Both cats became nervous and anxiously approached the window. The thing is that seeing them perform the customary ritual, I also knew that she was about to arrive. Suddenly, an uproar came from the street. I heard yells of accusation from the neighbors, and cries from Mi Niña, asking them to leave her alone. It didn't seem like they were assaulting her, just harassing, but it was the last straw. I took the first blunt object I found and rushed to go down to the street to defend her. I didn't get very far. From the stairs, the shouts were no longer heard. I didn't even get down one landing. What am I doing? I thought bewildered. That was already a loss of control, and I couldn't afford that. This could not be happening. It had to be a mistake. Resisting my urges, I turned and went back home. I remained standing, with my hands resting on the living room table, my head down, in a state of tremendous turmoil, my legs and arms shivering, until, slowly, I calmed down.

Bonita arrived home shortly afterwards. No one had assaulted her, no one had even addressed her, everything had occurred inside my mind. Again, it should have been irrefutable evidence that I needed medical treatment. But, once more, it wasn't. However, it served to keep me alert so that I never lost my temper again about something like that. It didn't matter what I could hear, what I thought was happening. Unless I saw things happen before my very eyes, nothing was going on. It was only this way that I could keep my actions under control. I felt that putting myself in someone else's hands would be fatal, the ultimate defeat. I was felt it instinctively, it was not a rational thrill. It came from my survival instinct, which, blatantly, was also altered. I didn't want to see me prostrate and sedated, perhaps locked up. I recalled over and over again the movie *One Flew Over the Cuckoo's Nest*. I did not want to end up like that.

The incident also served to make the voices take me more seriously, or be even madder at me, which is the same kind of thing. Thus, what was a regular neighborhood – though overzealous of its tranquility – was about to receive new signings to carry out its particular and overacted struggle against me, the crime.

Gasparín…

A new sinister character made his star appearance. He would displace Mr Tantrum as the coryphaeus of the barbarian horde that racked me day and night. He was, or better claimed to be, nothing less than a member of one of the corps of law and order, the Civil Guard, and he was, besides, an officer. I've never known his rank, for he never mentioned it. I could never get it from him either, since my voices are highly reluctant to volunteer any personal data. It is impossible to get even their first name out of them. This one made the mistake of saying it, or, at least, giving me a name in response to my constant requests. I always demanded they identify themselves and tell me plainly who they were and what they wanted. His name, apparently, was Gaspar.

    I couldn't help the temptation. Like a revelation, I immediately found the perfect nickname for this character. I was an expert in cartoon characters; I knew them all. One of the classic ones is the sweet ghost-child named Casper. In the episodes dubbed in Latin America, the name 'Casper' was replaced by the diminutive 'Gasparín'. Furthermore, the name was uttered with quite a honeyed pitch. I thought it was the perfect nickname, as 'Gasparín' is also a diminutive of Gaspar. Both characters shared the same ghostly essence, and there was also the ridiculous counterpoint between their personalities. I spent plenty of time dying of laughter. In an instant I had ruined the terrifying illusion of this fearful character, his careful staging. None of them ever dared to tell me their name from then.

    Gasparín was frightening and ruthless. He was the epitome of a tyrant. His stern and martial voice boomed out of nowhere like a whiplash, like a shot, shocking me. He did not speak, he gave categorical orders. One felt compelled to stand to attention even when he said good morning. He was Lt-Col. Tejero, he was Sgt Fury, he was Mussolini, he was Attila himself. He was all of them at once. I also sometimes called him 'Torrente' (an ugly, filthy, disgusting, and corrupt pseudo-cop character from a Spanish film), since I tirelessly worked to turn him into a mere clown. I was trying to wipe out the possible influence that such a terrible and fierce character could have on me. I used the ancient and effective method of deriding the opponent. It partly worked, but it was impossible to escape completely from his siege, from the effect of his repulsive voice, which exhaled profound scorn. There was a new sheriff in town. The law had come.

But Gasparín was not there on an official mission. His sense of responsibility had forced him to intervene as a simple citizen. Still, by no means did he stop exhibiting his status as an outstanding member of the Civil Guard, his status as an authority. Obviously, I never saw him or his badge, so I hadn't any reason to believe his word about his alleged status and rank. After all, impersonating the police is a fairly common trick when one wants to scare or impress someone, especially children. The image these blokes had of me was not exactly that of a respectable adult, so they could easily be using this trite childish trick to intimidate me.

At least they fitted the profile of the sort of people from whom I could expect such a simplistic hoax. Treating me like a child could also be an example of the refinement of his studied and obsessive desire to disturb and humiliate me. I used to spend a lot of time thinking about all the possibilities of this, trying to disentangle any logic that I was able to find in this mishmash of absurdities. The barrage was persistent and virulent. It was a psychological war, where defeat meant going mad or becoming incapacitated. My only option was to repel his attacks. I knew that I couldn't hurt him. I had no other choice, and that, in a sense, made me feel calm and secure. The decision was imposed on me: I had to resist.

The point is that the appearance of a lawman added possibilities to the situation. I was sure that the actions my stalkers were taking against me were blatantly lawless. Presenting themselves as bearers of justice, waving their police status as a banner, was the height of arrogance. In the field of logic and coherence, I had the upper hand. I guessed that this could be a cause of vexation for my bluenose hypocrite enemies. Why, if they were so right, didn't they just snitch on me to the real justice to settle the issue in court, as it should have been? I urged them to do so; I challenged them to do it. I wanted it all to end, but there was no way. I annoyed them by saying that they were the actual criminals. However, all my victories were pyrrhic. My self-confidence was strengthened, but the strikes on me were redoubled in counterpart. My persistent flouting barely made a dent in their self-esteem but it increased their thirst for revenge.

Gasparín used to appear and disappear like the little bird of a cuckoo clock. He had important business, aside from riling me, and was regularly absent, sometimes for many hours. Indeed, he had a kind of fixed schedule: a period in the morning and a period in the afternoon. Always more or less at the same time. Suddenly, his sounding voice would explode in my ear, and he would get on my nerves again. "I was pulling some strings," he would say – "and soon, I am going to do away with you."

He was trying to gather evidence, with the help of technology now. The hideous bugaboo did not hesitate in borrowing surveillance equipment from the police department to install around, on the roofs and rooftops. My flat was again being watched by a thousand eyes. Gasparín and his henchmen swarmed the rooftops, always invisible. In this way, they could go from spying on the front of my apartment to watching the back in seconds. They were trained men; they all knew their craft. My marijuana plantation and its attached lab would soon be uncovered, and I would end up in the hoosegow. I, for my part, questioned whether the evidence obtained illegally would be of any use to him, but there was nothing I could do, they went on stubbornly.

On their tours around the heights, they planted heaven-knows-what surveillance gadgets. Devices as invisible as their owners. They knew how to do their job. There was no way to detect them. I even placed two mirrors, which I found on the street, on both sides of my workroom window to have a panoramic view of the surroundings at a glance. In the living room, I put up an alarm with a presence detector, bought in a supermarket. They could try to storm my home through the false ceiling, which was accessible from the attic located above my apartment. I had to be prepared, you know.

I used to spend long hours working out on my gizmos, sitting on the floor in front of the window with mirrors, dividing my attention between working and stalking through my rudimentary counter-surveillance system.

On the right, my small marijuana plantation, on the left, one of my several computers. I used it to practice the piano with a midi keyboard. There was no lack of activities to occupy my long hours alone – okay, okay, almost alone. It was on one of those days I discovered, horrified, looking at the monitor of this particular computer, that I had made a big mistake. The plantation and its lighting were reflecting on the screen! The screen would be visible from the tops of many buildings on the street! At least, using binoculars or a telescope. Gasparín let me know, triumphant, with his deep martial voice and crushing assurance, that I was done. The local police had been warned and would soon arrive. Wow! So, after all this deployment, all this paraphernalia, weeks of relentless persecution, it was not going to be the Special Forces who would assault my home. He had called the local yokels, the city kitties. As if I had parked in his private parking spot. Wait! Of course, he could not mobilize his own men; his activities were clandestine, and his evidence was illegal. Everything had to seem normal; a casual discovery by a neighbor.

Instantly I put all my intellectual resources to work, trying to find a solution to the problem. My brain was on fire. I quickly studied every corner of the apartment, trying to find a new location for the damned plants. And I found it. The only place left out of prying eyes was the closet room. There was a gap between the wall and the wardrobes. The door with the fluorescent tubes which covered the plantation would fit without any problem. There was only one 'small' hindrance: this place was full of kitchen furniture, which in turn was full of stuff.

How I worked that afternoon! Put the plants in the interior room to get them out of sight, empty the kitchen furniture to be able to move it, remove it from the workroom, remove the door from the wall, take out the fluorescent tubes and the system of pipes for the carbon dioxide, make a hole in the door to install a fan – since there was no window to let the heat out – drill the wall, drill the side of the cabinet to install hardware to support the door, mount the fan, reassemble the fluorescent lights, put the door in place, put the plants below it, remove the timer that turns the lights on and off, install it in the inner room, put the kitchen cabinets where the plants were before, put all the junk back inside them, turn on the lights. And that was it, it was done. I was pouring with sweat and my hands ached from screwing and unscrewing so much and so quickly.

The police officers took their time. Gasparín and company waited for them on the edge of their seats, watching helplessly as their thwarted plan went up in smoke as time passed and the cops did not arrive. Moments after completing the move, when we all thought that the cops were not going to appear, they finally showed up. I could see in the window the unmistakable reflection of the blinking blue lights. I could hear the characteristic noise of their transmitters. I could also hear the engines of their motorcycles stopping in the street, in front of my door. And they were real, they were actually there, I could see them. They entered the building opposite. They were not going to my home, but to Gasparín's. They were all gathered there, trying to explain to the officers what had happened. The policemen, with an attitude that I found very professional, and in strict observance of the law, said that in my home there was nothing to see but a dude working on who knew what – I, of course, made it look like I was working, pretending not to be aware of anything. The cops said that there was no evidence of any illegal activity there, and they commanded them to stop spying on neighbors. I felt relieved and elated. In the end, it had blown up in their faces. Take that, Gasparín! Long live the municipal police! There would be more episodes like this.

That's how the plants ended up in their final location, locked in the junk room. The door to the room would only be opened to enter or exit, to avoid the suspicious glow emitted from inside. It looked like a door to another dimension. On the wall, behind the plants, I put up a poster of the movie *Torrente, el brazo tonto de la ley* (the silly arm of the law). It would be my last laugh if Gasparín ever came to see the infamous plantation with his own eyes. Sometime later, I also had to install some metal sheets on the wall. Gasparín got – I don't know where – an infrared whatchamacallit which allowed him to see through the walls. I used to spend a lot of time locked in that room, where I thought they couldn't see me. But it was clear that they could. It was only possible if they had such technology. He must have had military friends. It was too sophisticated and costly. How could they lend it out for such nonsense? This villain had no limits. He was entirely out of control.

... & Company

Apart from Mr Tantrum, the relentless Gasparín was not alone. He appeared surrounded by many other characters that were taking shape over time. In the first place, there were their relatives, since, after all, he was just one more neighbor. Gasparín was married, and his wife was a good woman, but as stereotypical as her husband. Gasparín's wife did not like what her icky husband and his cronies were doing. She often stepped in, trying to convince them to forget about the whole thing. She said that I was an ordinary person, that I earned my money working, that what they were doing was not right. She used to say it in a conciliatory tone, as though she were his grandmother. This spoiled the ominous and threatening effect of such a despotic community. It was as though Tejero's wife – the lieutenant colonel of the Civil Guard who tried to carry out the putsch on 23 February 1981, in Spain – had gone to the Congress in the middle of the 'Tejerazo' to urge him back home, saying that that was enough partying. Although they seemed to respect her, she never succeeded. She could only temporarily soften the mood of the horde. But they quickly got heated again, resuming their attacks. This character soon disappeared, which reinforced Gasparín's anger. Gasparín said that his wife had left him. She had walked out, and I was the culprit, of course. To put it mildly, he wasn't a very objective guy. Thus, the conflict became a personal matter for him, to which more and more offenses were added.

Gasparín's marriage had been fruitful. The harsh Mandarin had a daughter, a young woman who also served in the Civil Guard. Like her father, she had some officer rank, albeit lower than her father's. The wench was about to get married. Her bounteous father had bought her and her future husband an apartment. This flat was in the building opposite me, and it was still being renovated. It also faced the street, like mine. I was never able to discover its exact situation.

This character never had a name, at least not for me. She was just Gasparín's daughter. The voices did not appear to have the need to use names. They seemed to know who was addressing who, as if they were all in the same place together. For his daughter, Gasparín was, of course, just Dad. The rest of the voices, however, also ended up calling him Gasparín. If they ever used a name, they did it with the one I gave them, as a code name. The daughter played an ambivalent role in the story. On the one hand, she was as much an enemy of mine as her father. On the other hand, she often played a kind of moderating role, more in line with the idiosyncrasy of her generation, which must have been the same as mine.

Gasparín's daughter seems to have been the one who encouraged the rest of them to start this peculiar campaign against me. She did not want her children to grow up seeing activities like mine, to be victims of bad influences. "I want him out of the neighborhood!" Gasparín often used to spit out with his scornful voice. Perhaps that was the reason why the girl felt somehow responsible for the overzealousness of her enthusiastic advocates. Her future husband was, on the other hand, a friendly guy. He never joined the gang, and was always opposed to such an ugly affair. Sometimes, the planned wedding even appeared to be in danger. Maybe, this also fed the more moderate side of his future wife. After a time, he ended up breaking the engagement and disappeared forever. She was, for some time, very angry with me and then ended up fading away forever, as well. I am not a male chauvinist, in fact, I hate machismo, but on many occasions, when she intervened, I used to send her to go and do the dishes. It was too tempting. The rest of the machos used to laugh at the jibe, of course. All is fair in love and war. That annoyed her a lot, and I needed ammo, whatever it was.

Gasparín also seemed to have a son. A cheeky and unfriendly teenager; a worthy son of his father. I was unclear whether he was his real son or was only pretending to be to sound more impressive. Gasparín seemed to accept it as such, although without much enthusiasm. Sometimes he was his son, and sometimes he was not, as if that were one more tease, some kind of strategy to confuse me. In any case, it didn't matter. This was another character to whom I also gave a name. Since I often called his father Torrente, his unpleasant offspring was renamed 'Torrezno' (which, in Spanish, means both 'Torrente's cub' and 'fried bacon'). I always kicked him out. I had enough trouble with the adult vandals to have to deal with beardless children. His character was never very successful. He was just a ridiculous little boy who joined the oppressive chorus of voices without adding any substance to it. But the teen persisted in his pose. The truth is that the adult voices often silenced the minors – there were others – telling them not to get involved in men's business. The 'men' term referred to them, not to me, of course. They reproached me, in a somewhat hypocritical way, for the bad example I was giving to their tender infants: "Don't you realize that there are children present?" Everything served as an excuse to attack me.

There was also another renovation being carried out on Gasparín's flat. This added to the fearsome and spooky legion a new gang of quarrelsome workers. They were headed by a brutal foreman whom I imagined tall and robust, according to the image suggested by his voice. I mentally drew him with a thick black beard and – I don't know why – a horizontal striped white and blue T-shirt, like a sailor's. I could never find a ridiculous enough nickname for him. I tried 'Budespencer', referring to the well-known actor, noted for his terrible fists. I tried 'Don Pimpón', a monstrous farmer with bulging and bloodshot eyes, from the Spanish version of *Sesame Street*. I also tried '*el Barbas*' (the Beard). It was simpler, albeit not very witty. He was one of Gasparín's strongest and most courageous allies, with whom the abject campaign leadership was disputed. A dark consulate that kept me constantly besieged for almost two years.

A citizen with Gasparín's status, with his peculiar interpretation of the legality and the prerogatives of his position, couldn't but have a private attorney. Gasparín's lawyer followed with concern the covert operations of such a snooping troop. He used to warn him of the flagrant breaches contrary to the law that they were perpetrating. His warnings were ever unheeded by his rampant client. The sins of the sinners will be later forgiven by the priest. Gasparín would be later released from jail by his attorney. Nothing could stop the zeal of such a despicable and devoted hound. *Dura lex, sed lex*. Especially when he was the law.

The different police forces usually cooperate with each other, each according to its competences and jurisdictions. I don't quite remember how, but the National Police soon joined the crusade. I guess they were Gasparín's friends or acquaintances. He invited them to contemplate and comment on his work, trying at the same time to gain new allies. It seems that, just being a half-mad drug addict, I was being a tough nut to crack. Again, I deduced they had police status from the pitch and timbre of their voices, less martial than Gasparín's military voice, but transmitting authority, along with that careful technical indifference that only the police has.

Of course, they weren't just police officers, they had to have been at least inspectors, even a commissioner. There were not many, maybe two or three; I never managed to count my voices. The one who appeared to be a commissioner initially interceded on my behalf. Not in my defense, but as if giving me a chance to depose my attitude peacefully, submitting to unknown twisted designs. To my mind, I couldn't see what I had to do to compensate for such a display of means, such an annoyance, so much bile shedding, so much humiliation of such superior beings, and so many offenses. Had I just to relinquish my few plants, which were nothing more than a whim? Had I to turn myself in to the authorities, to receive as punishment a small fine, or probably not even that, given my mental condition? That was a dead end. The classic good cop/bad cop game didn't stick. I stubbornly refused to follow even the most innocuous advice, so this cop also ended up siding with my most bitter enemies. This new haunter added the resources of the National Police to those of the Civil Guard. Cops worthy of the vilest banana republic, if all this really had happened. What would I have to do in the face of such formidable enemies? Even if I got evidence, would I risk reporting it? I could end up buried in quicklime somewhere far away.

The army couldn't be missing in that bunch. They were two, only appearing once in a while, and they were the meanest of them all. Their threats were of death and torture and they even threatened to rape Mi Niña. I think sometimes they even horrified the others, who asked them to calm down a bit. I had to be careful about offending them. But I always ended up exasperating everybody, owing to my reactions while I was taking the flak. They told me what their rank was: "We are *brigadas* (sgt major) of the Spanish Army." They were proud of it, and they were not afraid of anything or anyone. I was quite surprised by the fact that they were '*brigadas*', since it is a rank that I would never have used for a character of my invention. Sergeants, lieutenants, captains, but '*brigadas*'? They couldn't have come from my imagination. They didn't use my vocabulary. They made mistakes that I would not make. Undoubtedly, we are more than capable of completely deceiving ourselves.

At times, I joked about so much diversity: "You only lack the priest, the bullfighter and the flamenco dancer." "Surely you look like The Village People." There were also other secondary folk who were less sinister that we could call 'the minor voices'. These were closer to what a real person would be. You already know Mr Tantrum. He was the stereotype of the cranky old man who is always angry. There was, and he is still around here, a severe and circumspect old man who frequently repeated to me, "Change your attitude!". He wasn't threatening or aggressive. He didn't seem a mean person, but he was a busybody and as persistent as the others, although he tried not to go too far. He used to say that I was quite an insolent because of my outbursts and the gross words I used for them. "Well, look there now. The high and mighty sir thinks I am insolent. What they do is the most normal thing ever." I owed them respect, apparently. I always sent him packing. Sometimes I called him '*Don Senén*' or '*Don Homobono*'; nothing rude.

There was 'Mr Levamos', to whom I gave this name one day when he was releasing a litany of threats, all of them beginning with the expression '*Le vamos a*' (we are going to…): "We are going to do this to him, we are going to do that to him!" Mr Levamos' voice was more like that of a clerk, an office worm, though not a book one. He didn't seem like a tough guy, not even a bully. He was more like a big softy. For this reason, his threats sounded ridiculous and implausible. He was more like the one who receives the punches than who gives them. Maybe that's why he used the plural instead of the singular, as I once pointed out to him. He felt emboldened and became presumptuous among so much bouncer.

There were a few more of these little puppies attached to the pack of mastiffs, there always are, but they were not actually a problem, as they did not really impress me very much. Indeed, some small foe like this gave me satisfaction now and then. They were almost a blessing, a bagatelle.

I nicknamed another '*El Amiguete*' (the Homeboy). He seemed to be a middle-aged man, and his attitude was friendly, as his name suggests. He appeared to be sincere and used to cheer me up and advise me to be brave so that the others would stop hassling me. He did not urge me to do or stop doing anything. He was a friend, or at least an acquaintance, from the rest of the voices. None of the others messed with him for his attitude. He was a normal guy, he was totally free to make decisions, even contrary to the rest. That was one of the things that I was supposed to learn to do: I had to act before them like a real man, to treat the matter seriously.

From my side, I didn't feel motivated to integrate into a community like that. That mob wanted to appropriate, by force, a deal that I thought was just my own business. If I yielded to their intolerable pressures, I would enter the group as a humiliated and subdued member, a subordinate. It did not seem the best position from which to fraternize, or the most convenient way to enter into a bargain of any kind. "No negotiation with terrorists," I replied. One doesn't negotiate with a gun on the table. They laughed: "But do you think that people like us were going to negotiate with someone like you?" This method was used often: "But do you think we...?" Every time I thought I'd understood what they wanted from me they racked me about it for fun. "In any case," I replied, "you act as if you wanted something from me. It is clear that I have something that you want, and you have nothing to offer me in exchange." No, I was not going to fall into their trap. They were rabble, and I wasn't going to let them trample on me. I was not going to make any concessions to them. When they believed me defeated, on the verge of crumbling, Gasparín used to ask, in a triumphant and resonant voice: "Are you willing to bear the consequences of your actions?" The answer was always, "Go fuck yourselves."

They're the Emotions, Stupid!

I suppose it is hard to believe that someone can take as real the vaudeville that I have just described. It is utterly crazy, extravagant, grotesque, and ridiculous. But the voices besieged me endlessly, and even now still do, at times. The voices take turns, taking over from one another. They give no quarter. If I manage to take control of the fight with one of them, somehow neutralizing his attack, others come to his aid or substitute him. The content, as they tell me, is not as relevant as the way and the moment it is said. It seems that one is in the hands of a group of expert torturers, who work tirelessly day and night. It doesn't matter what time I wake up; there they are, even in dreams. It is funny, in dreams, they behave the same way as they do when I'm awake. They are neither more nor less absurd.

We are social beings. Our mind has been shaped by evolution to respond emotionally to the interactions with others. We can even get excited with simple objects that remind us of human beings. We can feel tenderness before the sweet little face, studiously modeled, of a doll. We can feel a tickle of sexual excitement by observing statues in sexually-explicit positions, even looking at simple drawings with pornographic scenes. We have created a whole gallery of imaginary monsters that make us uneasy or scared when we hear stories about them. We can make up or deform our faces in such a way that we cause fear, disgust, or laughter. Our gestures transmit all kinds of emotions, and we know how to fake them to delude others. We play with our voice's tone and inflections to better report about our thoughts, our intentions, and our personality.

All this shapes the complex phenomenon that we know as 'empathy'. It is even known that there is a type of specialized neuron for it, the so-called 'mirror neurons'. Empathy allows us to internalize others and decipher, on the basis of our own emotions and feelings, the emotions and feelings of others. We can even empathize with other species, insofar as they transmit understandable messages to us that we can translate into human emotions. By experiencing what goes through another's mind, we can feel sorry for him, fear him, love him, and, of course, hate him.

Language, which is perhaps the most human of our characteristics, is also one of the most potent manipulation tools available to us. A fundamental principle is etched deep in our minds. A principle that automatically assaults us with a visceral sense of conviction, preparing us for possible interaction: if something speaks, then it is human. We humans do not just help one another, we also compete and fight for resources. Our most fearsome enemies are amongst the members of our own species. Naturally, we have a knee-jerk alarm signal that immediately warns us of the presence of another person in the vicinity, addressing us: "Beware: human!"

I am a tremendously realistic person, as incredible as it sounds. Although perhaps I enjoy an overflowing fantasy, under normal conditions I can separate it without any problem from reality. For that reason, my voices were, and still are, people. Judgement and reason can modulate the emotional response over the most visceral animal reactions, for instance, realizing that you are being teased or watching a play. When listening to the voices, one can change the instinctive thrills caused by the situation, but only up to a point, for new feelings immediately rise as new interactions occur.

A continuous hammering of powerful stimuli causes our attention to get tired, our mental defenses to weaken, and consciousness to lose control of the situation. This is known and used by all interrogators. If one hears someone speak to them with great anger, even if they don't understand the speaker's language, one has a gut reaction to the emotion directed at them. If the other's pitch indicates that they are about to attack, one already feels threatened just because of this, no matter what the other is saying.

But they can also use sophisticated and Machiavellian techniques of mental manipulation to exhaust all the resources of one's mind until one gives in. A common one is switching between attack and a friendly attitude. Continual mood shifts, too, cause one's brain to produce different substances and use various neural networks until all the reserves are drained. The well-known game of good cop, bad cop is based on this. They can add belittling and humiliation, which, likewise, generate strong emotions and feelings. First, I scare you, then, I laugh at your fear, then, I reassure you; I make fun of you again for thinking that I can feel sympathy for you, and so it goes on endlessly. The goal is to induce debilitating feelings: fear, helplessness, despair. It is about breaking one's defenses, crumbling one's mental walls, getting one to surrender, and submitting one's will. It is like the poliorcetics ancient art: the art of conducting and resisting sieges of cities and strongholds.

Hate is a hellish instrument against people. Hate, like love, is one of the strongest feelings, a binding emotion. Like love, hatred creates an indelible bond with the hated person. Hate consumes one's resources and weakens reason, making one act thoughtlessly. If our enemies get us to hate them, they place a torpedo on our waterline. Hate is like the Trojan horse: *Timeo Danaos et dona ferentes*, 'I fear the Greeks even when they bear gifts'. It is very tempting to feel it, but it always takes its toll. Never allow yourself to feel hatred for your enemies. It is a survival tip that I hope you never need.

The voices attacked using all sorts of trickery, although there were also a few resting periods. Sometimes, it seemed that they'd got sick of the matter, and they would let it be for a while, as if saying that they were in control, that for them it was just a kind of hobby. They were showing a poor intelligence. Wit is not necessary, because achieving the feeling of oppression takes no intellectual effort. Showing themselves as assholes is even an exercise of studied sadism, one further humiliation. For my part, the strategy was to avoid socializing with the voices at all costs and prevent creating emotional bonds with them. I had to despise, to belittle, to ignore them. I had to try and nullify them to neutralize the effect that the admonitory, aggressive, or taunting intonations had on me. But also their friendly attitude. I had to delete them from my list of peers, of human beings.

Oddly enough, the voices apparently cooperated in some way on the project. They sabotaged their own attempts by sneering at me at the slightest sign of hesitancy. They seemed so eager to lay me low that they were beyond the ridiculous. I always tried to see the funny side, me making fun of them, too. But I had to be careful of this, to be objective, not insulting, and not to be a big-mouth. It wasn't about offending at any cost. Any blunder would end up embarrassing me and turning against me.

Luckily, my voices offered enough opportunities for me to make fun of them – and rightly so. They suffered from immense pettiness, as well as vast stupidity. They deserved it. That undermined their possible power over me while reinforcing my self-confidence when I was successful. But I couldn't always laugh at the situation or at them as my mood was not always favorable. Their counter-attacks could break my defensive lines and drive me back to states of anguish and depression. I spun nonstop on an emotional maelstrom, on a soul roller coaster, hitting and being hit. I remember being cringed in a corner of the dinette on one occasion, crying desperately in silence, all the home lights turned off and the blinds down, while the voices incessantly harassed me. Fortunately, I soon overcame that initial weakness.

Those voices did not have a human counterpart, a real body or face. This entailed a lack of relevant information in my mind. The most distinctive voices, like Gasparín's, were perfectly recognizable, but others were blurred, and they mixed in such a way that I could not differentiate between them. The voices took advantage of this fact and played a kind of misleading game, in which one feigned to be another. They told me that each of them could make several different voices, even asserting that there was only one person (perhaps me?) who spoke, faking all the voices and personalities. They used to say that they were only teasing me, and they often repeated it. At the same time, the hostility and the feelings against me seemed utterly sincere. All of this fueled the fire of my confusion. We were playing a perverse game: resistance or serfdom, a duel of wills.

"Ignore them"; "to foolish words, deaf ears…" We can learn all the tag lines and idioms we want but none of them will work. One has to learn how not to feel. It is not enough to believe that it is better not to do it; it is not even enough to be sure about it. Visceral emotions, just as a heartbeat, cannot be controlled with simple arguments. Reason and the heart are in separate body areas; different jurisdictions. I think that reason is itself a complex and sophisticated aggregate of fine-grained thrills. But probably the interference between reason and the most basic emotional tiers is suboptimal. On those levels, reactions must be quick. Reason is slow, but very good at analyzing, correlating, investigating, judging, and drawing conclusions. It has access to the outer and our inner worlds. By reasoning, we can learn how to use the environment to influence our internal state, and assign certain connotations to words, objects, deeds, etc. We can learn that performing certain actions produces certain feelings, and how to combine some of these feelings to build others. Reason is more a counselor than a leader.

Hallucinations and delusions are positive symptoms of psychosis. They are something that shouldn't be there. There are also negative symptoms, personality traits that decrease or disappear. One can become asocial, withdrawing from others, and lose interest in interacting with them. I am neither too sociable nor too asocial a man and this did not seem to be altered. Anhedonia is the loss of the ability to take pleasure in what one does. I did not experience anhedonia whatsoever. I liked and enjoyed doing many things, almost manically. Avolition is the loss of will. My will remained firm, even in excess; it seemed to me that my life depended on it. Alogy is the loss of fluency in speech. Sometimes, the voices would get in the way, and I could lose track of the conversations, that's true, but I don't think my ability for expression was affected either. I needed language to defend myself; it was essential to me. The affective flattening consists of the decrease or disappearance of emotional reactions. One feels indifferent to the people or events in one's environment. I did suffer from this, albeit selectively. I could feel intensely emotions that reinforced my ability to face the voices, making me feel good. But those that could become a weakness seemed to fade away.

A friend of ours was unexpectedly diagnosed with a very aggressive cancer. He was admitted to hospital until his death, a short time later. We often came to visit him, and we saw him getting worse day by day. I couldn't feel anything for him. I was incapable. I knew what I was supposed to feel, and I wanted to feel it, but there was no emotion. On one occasion, Mi Niña, who is asthmatic, got the flu. It affected her lungs so virulently she could barely breathe. We went to the doctor immediately. I was indifferent. I wasn't worried about the situation. I couldn't understand it. I was flummoxed and acted like a robot, like it was nothing. Later, I had to call a taxi to take her to the hospital urgently. I still felt nothing. She was admitted to the ICU, and I had to go home because I was also starting to show flu symptoms. This loss worried me much more than the voices themselves. I seemed to have repressed these kinds of debilitating emotions as a defense mechanism; as if all my emotional endowment was being invested in my inner war.

Happily, Bonita recovered, and the episode was never repeated. For me, the lack of pain and worry in these situations was a loss of an essential part of my life. I wish I had suffered, paradoxical as it may be. They will always constitute a hole in my existence, something that should have been there but was not. It was a negative symptom in every way.

In a situation like mine, it is not that one loses contact with reality. Such a situation is not perceived as wholly incredible. Reality is still there. The plot and its characters also seemed absurd to me. I was able to reason that they couldn't be real, but it didn't matter: I felt like they were real, period. The pressure, plus the intoxication, was preventing me from not only thinking but feeling clearly. My reasoning was in pretty good shape. It allowed me to work, carefully plan my actions, my strategies, doubt my senses, and study my enemies in great detail. Even so, my emotional state did not allow me to reject the situation as impossible, to stop consuming narcotics, to seek some type of treatment instead of engaging in a dicey fight with more than dubious results.

To Infinity, But Not Beyond

The voices could act as a team of psychological maulers, but they were able to set a limit on their abuses. One day, amid an overwhelming storm of voices, who harried me in a fierce chorus, I thought I recognized my father's voice among them. It was like a blast, discovering my father allied with such a gang of motherfuckers. I didn't understand anything. I felt nonplussed and began to cry disconsolately, gasping and babbling, asking for both apologies and explanations.

Then, the voices had me where they wanted. But their reaction was surprising. All of a sudden, they stopped their blitz and began to reassure me. They insisted that it was not my father, that I got confused. They talked among themselves, stressing that they couldn't go down such a road. Their tone was that of someone who has crossed the line unwittingly and wants to back down. It was just that the voice of one of them could be confused with my father's, though it was not alike if I had really paid attention. The air cleared, the harassment was suspended for a while, and I calmed down and recovered. I never confused them again.

The voices never said a dirty word either. They called me delinquent, something that I took as an exaggeration rather than an insult. They called me drug addict, something that was true and to which I responded with, "Tell me something I don't know". But they never insulted me or my family or friends. If they ever tried, it became clear that they were not used to it. Neither the vilest among them, nor the biggest bullies, or the most opinionated, or those who seemed most stupid, ever released a swear word.

Their language could be quite limited, but, in that sense, they seemed polite people. They could lie or threaten, but not insult.

Unlike the voices, I do not refrain from saying rude things, mouthing off expletives, swearing in Aramaic, or even blaspheming if the situation requires it. One of my high school literature teachers used to tell us in class that a cultured person is the one who knows how to behave appropriately in any situation. I liked the sentence so much, and it appeared so right to me, that I adopted it as a motto. It's about adding, not about selecting. You have to expand yourself in all possible directions. I love language; it could be said it fascinates me. I am passionate about it. I can use the language of logic, of mathematics, the language of computers. I have even designed some programming language. I can speak to educated people, but I can also go unnoticed in an inadvisable dump, expressing myself in prison slang. Let's talk to each person in their own language.

This was another conundrum that made me doubt my authorship of the voices. It is not that insults and profanity impress me particularly, but used with some insistence, they can be effective. The use of rich language serves to convey a certain sense of authority. Playing with the meaning is superior only to playing with the intonation. If you combine both possibilities, the result can be the perfect rhetoric. Why use weak and simplistic logic for making the voices, if you have a better repository of knowledge? They were only successful in annoying me. Rather than pretending to bring me down psychologically, they were bent on 'making me jumpy'. They often used to repeat it. But they were at once too simplistic. I could create more sophisticated and compelling characters. When the voices were those of my co-workers or my family, they were indistinguishable from their real models, who were not at all stupid. I suppose the explanation is that they were primarily made based on stereotypes. They were the kind of stereotypes that highlight negative aspects and ridicule or criminalize a group of people. Perhaps this way it was more humiliating. Maybe I am quite Machiavellian.

Sometimes, it appeared that I could also, in a way, take control of the voices for a while. More than controlling the originals, I was able to create kind of clones that, with some effort, I could make say what I wanted. The actual voices were hidden by these bogus voices, who only spoke rubbish or repeated a single word over and over again. Their task was nothing other than to mask the real voices. It was not that I felt these false voices were something I was doing consciously. In part, they also seemed alien to me, though they were undoubtedly under my control. The effect was similar to when you talk nonsense out loud so that you can't hear what someone is saying to you. By using bhang, it was even easier to get it.

The marijuana that grew at home was not just ornamental. Although I didn't smoke a lot, I always had a little joint at night with which to go to bed. Then, the voices used to protest endlessly, threatening me, and speaking about me with contempt. In response, I sometimes created clones to shush them and changed them for a sort of monk or priest of some esoteric cult performing an absurd and ridiculous ritual. "We are the major arcana," they assured me in a serious and pompous tone. Next, they began to take turns emitting a kind of muffled esoteric chant with soft 'poms' and 'fuuss' sounds uttered with the greatest reverence. I imagined them dressed in robes and playing fanciful instruments. I couldn't hold back the laughter, it was so ridiculous.

Suddenly, one of them would mimic a firework rocket sound as they ascended: "Shhhhhhh." Then, also with much reverence, another would emit a long, muffled "boooom". And back again. When I was already writhing with laughter in bed, internally – Bonita was next to me – everything would stop, like a bubble bursting. The voices ceased to be the major arcana and went back to being the major whoresons. And they went wholly ballistic! What an anger they held! They felt very offended and tremendously insulted. And then would begin a virulent attack of angry voices. Laughter gave way to oppression. I learned how to relax, get the rebuke to draw away, and lower the voices gradually.

Again, it was a Pyrrhic victory. The price to pay was quite high. It was not a good technique, but it spoiled the feeling of realism. This happened at the beginning of this third episode, when I wondered what or who would be the new voices that I heard everywhere. Once their personalities were defined, I couldn't repeat this again. Did this convince me that the voices were a product of my mind? No, never completely. I just believed that I was mixing hallucinations with a real situation. Honestly, at that time, I was convinced that they were in my neighborhood, that they were flesh and blood people. My paranoia did not allow me to rule it out, despite the fact that I already knew from experience that it was possible to superimpose auditory hallucinations on what was actually being said around me.

An undecidable proposition is that which one cannot prove or disprove. Instead of truth, one has to use beliefs. The truth, the facts, are not chosen, but the beliefs are. Belief and certainty are emotionally very similar, if not entirely the same. Certainty is only the highest degree of belief. Our minds are always littered with undecidables and hypotheses. In a state of emotional disturbance, we can come to accept almost anything as possible. The feeling is the same as when one is in a normal state. People with mental disorders don't believe differently, only in different things.

Regardless of the fact that some of them seemed to side with me at times, I decided that the best and simplest strategy was to consider them all as foes. I was sorry if anyone acted in good faith, but the gloves were off. Even in these circumstances, I harbored a certain sympathy for those who behaved in a more moderate and civilized way. It was something like Stockholm syndrome. Either way, those were just as intrusive as the others. What could be called 'the good voices' would cause me nearly as many problems as those that assaulted me mercilessly, the 'mean voices'. With the bad guys, the corresponding reaction was much clearer. They did not feel any positive empathy towards other people. Neither did I towards them.

The thing is, I started not to make distinctions between them, and made fun of and rejected them all, sometimes even against my true feelings. I had to be hard. It was a war. There were only two sides, and on one of the sides there was only me, and it should only be me. I would not admit any defectors from the enemy. I was not going to accept possible traitors. I was going to give them reasons to really hate me. Mind your own business! After all, it could only be our self-esteem that was wounded. It didn't feel like there was going to be any physical violence.

A Million Followers

Such a gang of bloodhounds was not going to limit itself to simply stalking my home. Leaving home became a disturbing experience. I got the feeling that a thousand eyes were watching me. I heard countless voices around that sounded as if they were talking about me, about what I was doing, as though reporting it to someone else. The voices began to follow me beyond the limits of my block. Gasparín and his henchmen mobilized their underlings to give me no space anywhere. Sometimes, they even followed me down the street. But outdoors, I felt in a way safer than at home. At least there were witnesses all around.

The problem was how to know who was a witness and who was a haunter. They did their job very well. It could be said they were professionals. It was like being immersed in Bentham's panopticon, the utopian prison system: All prisoners could be watched day and night by their guards, unable to see them or know where they were, but always knowing that they were there, surveilling. I used to sneak a peek around, to find out who was muttering behind my back. I tried to detect some disregard, some gaze, or sign of any kind. I used the reflections in the windows and mirrors of the parked cars, in the storefronts, or in every other sort of glass panes. But the people around me, whether they were close or far away, were doing their own thing. No one seemed to notice me. Many times it was impossible to find out who was speaking. Many times there was no one in sight.

To be alone in the street, but feeling that I was being followed, and hearing comments about my actions, was a minor problem for me. I suffered from psychosis, paranoia, and persecutory delusions. I could listen out for them and then they were there, behind any object, a tree, for instance, or crouching behind or inside a car. Even inside a postbox. Everything was possible. There were also the houses along the street. After all, they were servants of the law. They just had to ring the bell, display their badge, and say something like: "Police on duty, we need to get into your home to monitor a suspect."

Eventually, the voices would come out from everywhere. Even impossible places, such as street bins, lamp posts, road signs, bollards… Anything around could suddenly start talking. Maybe they had hidden small speakers with a receiver to confuse me so that I couldn't locate them. There was always an explanation. Of course, I knew that my mental state was altered. I knew that the situation was impossible, although this wasn't irrefutable evidence that everything was inside my mind. I only accepted that part of it must have been. It was true that they followed me, but, in my state, I was not able to locate the origin of the voices. They seemed to come from impossible places. Both things were compatible. I struggled to find evidence and compelling reasons against these beliefs, but there was no way. I couldn't disregard them. I thought that, if I did, I would go back to normal. Everything else would disappear along with the beliefs.

Traveling by public transport was even worse than walking down the street. I usually don't take the bus as I prefer the subway. Sometimes, I had no choice but to use it. But it was not easy. There is a great concentration of people, plus a high level of background noise. Think about the shrill screeching of train brakes when entering the station. It can be a chilling experience for someone with altered perception and senses. It can be heard as usual, which is unpleasant enough, but it can also be an incredible rumble that seems to fill one up completely. It was an adrenaline high that shocked me – a bit like that dizziness when we get up suddenly, only a much more intense sensation. For me, it was also proof that my ears were extremely sensitive.

In return, the sound of the crowd's speaking masked what the voices were saying quite well, and, sometimes, it was a break. On my strolls, I also discovered that the sound of water from the great monumental fountains almost completely masked the chatter of the voices. I had tried headphones and white noise recording, but it was not very helpful and more annoying than anything else. I was determined to find a remedy. I had to know whether my persecutors existed or not.

Inside the train carriages, there is much less noise, or at least fewer voices speaking at once. There I could hear the mumbling of my chasers. Leaning against the wall at the end of the carriage, I had a complete view of its interior. I could sneakily observe all the travelers. There seemed to be comments about me coming from all the seats. There even appeared to be some speaking on the radio to report on me. But only when I wasn't looking. There was no way to catch them red-handed here, either. Maybe I could mislead them?

I recalled the famous scene of the chase in the movie *French Connection*. The sly drug dealer Alain Charnier dodges his tenacious persecutor, the dogged policeman nicknamed Popeye, in the New York Subway, with a series of skillful movements of entering and exiting the train carriages just before the doors start closing. *Well, let's try something like that*, I told myself. So I stood, relaxed, near the door, as if I wasn't going to get off at the next station. I waited for the doors to start closing and jumped out at the last minute. The convoy moved away, carrying my outwitted haunters. But, on the next train, I unavoidably had more of the same. They had definitely been tracking my movements through the surveillance cameras. They must have men at all stations. I didn't repeat the experiment many times. There was no way to escape the siege.

However, I did not deprive myself of going out. I was not afraid. I kept thinking that, on open ground, I would have the opportunity to unmask my stalkers, discover what they looked like, and eliminate part of my disadvantage by knowing something more about them. I knew that it was impossible to surmise a person's appearance just by hearing his voice. For me, Gasparín was a big, moustached guy, the stereotype of a civil guard, and I always imagined him in his uniform, including the tricorn. That didn't help much in locating potential candidates. I hadn't a defined physical image of the other voices, except perhaps for *el Barbas*, the chunky gaffer in charge of the renovation in the home of the evil *picoleto*. But he was just a mason or something like that. He never carried out any surveillance work. He was just a neighborhood bully who was up for any excuse and opportunity to abuse. *El Barbas* was only a problem at home.

From time to time I went to my old workplace. I would chat for a while with my brother, my former colleagues, and my bosses – who were still so, since they continued paying me despite my leave. My indefatigable persecutors always followed me there, of course. They even dared to go upstairs and try to convince A that I was a dangerous criminal and she had to collaborate with the authorities – them – to keep me off the streets. A's office was next to the front door. From the furthest part of the office, where almost everyone else worked, I could hear Gasparín trying to convince A vehemently. Meanwhile, she yelled expletives at him demanding, as a lawyer, to leave me in peace and to get the hell out immediately.

My former hallucinations faced the new ones. Gasparín always had to back down and leave with his tail between his legs. On the way out, I would pick him up and lead him back home, like a child with his balloons. They were stuck to the soles of my shoes like disgusting chewing gum balls, never showing their faces. All of them so powerful and at the same time such cowards. But they could still overcome their wickedness.

That Dirty Little Coward That Shot Mr. Howard

So far, the diatribes of the voices had been targeted solely at me. There were a few shy threats against Bonita, but I considered these like an outburst of rage. But, the wicked Gasparín, since his attacks were all unsuccessful, began to threaten to kill my dear cats, who were like my children. "I'm going to kill his cats!" he would spit in his despicable voice. Among the wide range of felonies that human beings can commit, those that I consider the most abhorrent are torture, rape, kidnapping, murder, and killing pets.

Once the Nazis had humiliated and forced out the Jews from their jobs and businesses, they went door to door, taking away their pets to kill them all because they were considered a nuisance. Later, they took their owners and killed them too. When I find these stories in novels, movies, or even history books, they always turn my stomach. Historical facts are the most terrible of all because they really happened. In particular, hurting the pets of those people who establish strong emotional ties with them is like causing harm to a loved one. Many people consider the love that we put into these kinds of relationships to be exaggerated: "It's just a dog!"; "It's just a cat!". He is only a son, she is only a sister, he is only a friend… Why stop at just animals? Are we more genetic than emotional? Who, honestly, gives a damn about genetics? Do you know or worry more about your genes than about your emotions?

This is a particularly sore point because society is so 'humanitarian' with people, even with the most execrable ones, but does not consider ending the life of one of these defenseless buddies to be a significant crime. It is not only an attack against an animal, but also a cruel act of aggression against a human being. The law is too soft to really protect pets. Killing my cats could cause me great pain, but, for them, it would just be fun. Absolute impunity. Surely it would be a more serious crime to shoot at the house than to kill two simple cats. Perhaps there would be a small fine, which they would pay, laughing in my face at the double humiliation: I killed your loved ones, and now, I am paying for them, as if they were just pieces of meat.

This was the definitive reason that made me feel a profound rejection and hostility towards such nauseating unwanted company. Even so, I didn't hate the voices. As I have said before, I was not going to establish a close bond with those disgusting beings. I was not going to allow them to be part of me. But the feeling of rejection towards them became absolute. I used to accuse the unworthy Gasparín of being devilish, demonic. He owned the weapon with which he intended to perpetrate such an abomination. It was with this that he mainly used to threaten. Even the Mafia had tried to establish, as a golden rule, that family should not be touched in a vendetta. My cats were innocent victims. I wasn't going to forgive a thing like that.

But there wasn't much I could do about it. I tried to explain to Mi Niña, diplomatically, that I believed that the neighbors' irritation could lead to them doing something against the cats. But she refused to have them locked in the interior part of the house. When I was alone with them, I used to take both in my lap when the voices spat their threats, sitting on the window sill, with my back facing outwards, as though challenging them to shoot me, too, in the back, like hitmen or terrorists. They proudly presented themselves as representatives of law and order. I thought that likening them to the most abject criminals would have some effect on their self-esteem, but they did not seem to care too much. Sometimes, a shy reproach arose among their ranks, but nothing significant. The fearsome mastiff was not going to let go of his prey so quickly. He wouldn't lose that opportunity, no matter how immoral it would be.

It was during this period that another one of the surprising coincidences that seemed to prove the reality of the surreal story I was living happened. One day, when I was back home, I found that the cats' water bowl was empty. It was hot, and for sure they were thirsty, so I went to fill it, as usual. Nothing came out from the tap. Gasparín had also recruited to his cause the mercenary gang of workers who carried out the renovation in my building. I did not have to wait long to hear his hateful voice proclaiming that he had cut off the water and that my cats could die of thirst, as far as he was concerned.

Gasparín's daughter commiserated, and begged him then not to be mean. She told him to let me give my kittens a drink, and just prevent me from drinking if what he wanted was to fuck me off. Gasparín reluctantly agreed, grumbling: "Okay, okay, now you can give your damn cats a drink!" Lo and behold I turned on the tap again, and there was the water. As soon as I refilled the bowl, the water was cut off anew. Nay, these things were not helpful to convince me that I was just delusional. Even if they only happened on very few occasions.

The silly brawl was taking on an outlandish tinge. I was besieged by countless hostile suckers over nothing. They were ready to commit all the baseness that they considered necessary. And just for the sake of a ragged and outdated morality that debased itself through such despicable defenders and methods. The end justifies the means. *Fiat iustitia et pereat mundus.* Again, I had to pluck up courage and risk the irreplaceable loss of my cats, trusting that what I believed was happening was not real at all, or that those unprincipled would not actually be so heartless. And, of course, the thing worked. Nothing bad ever happened to my cats. No one caused them any harm. Who was going to do it?

It is so hard to leave home thinking that it will be the last time you'll see your loved ones alive. Nevertheless, at the same time, it was an excellent school in overcoming fears, based on high doses of realism – exposure therapy. What does not kill you makes you stronger. Gradually, I was moving from being a timorous drug addict to face challenges – imaginary but nevertheless, still tough – of courage. But consumption continued. The idea of finally abandoning it often popped back into my head. It was not a pleasant thought and I procrastinated the thorny decision over and over again. I had other problems to solve first.

I tried to find ways to catch my elusive watchers by surprise. I bought a tiny video camera in an electronics store that I used to frequent. It was cheap, since it was only a plate with a lens to which I had to solder the cables to connect it to a play-recorder. Enthusiastically, I mounted the counter-surveillance device and set it up to obtain material evidence of the existence of those miserable neighbors. It goes without saying that the camera never recorded anything or anybody. No one on the roofs or on the balconies or at the windows. The videotapes did not have the capacity for much recording time either. The camera ended up in the junk pile once I got bored with it. I still keep it as a memory of such bizarre days.

The best way to overcome the helplessness is by achieving the sensation that you are not stopped, immobilized, or defeated. One has to do anything one can. I couldn't stop planning ideas and putting them into practice, no matter how crazy they seemed. It is good advice, of course, to be sure that such actions are not dangerous to anyone, but, apart from that, it is the best thing to do. As a well-known advertisement said: 'If you don't move, you become obsolete.'

After a while, they softened towards me when they realized how I was taking it all, saying from time to time that they were only fooling me and were not really going to do it. The voices had a fixation on that. It seemed that everything was allowed because they were only doing it 'to fool you'.

We Shall Fight on the Beaches

Any living being has fundamentally three options when facing a threat: escaping, remaining paralyzed to go unnoticed, or defending itself against danger. All three are valid, and the best choice depends on the situation and the circumstances. The 'evil voices' basically constituted aggression. The attackers have already seen you, they know who and where you are. Hiding is not an option. Escape is impossible, neither is it a valid option. It does not matter what the voices are, they will always be around you, or inside your head. The only option left, then, is self-defense. If one thinks about it, having a single option greatly facilitates decision making. The survival instinct, the determination to not be trampled and humiliated by anyone, and even self-esteem are the fuel that moves towards self-defense, but one has to get it ignited.

If one is an alpha individual, dominant by nature, one is way ahead of the game. I am alpha, and I am also Aries, a fire sign. Stubborn, rebellious, and aggressive, though not aggressor. Our planet is Mars, the god of war. I think aggression is a weakness of the spirit, but I see defense as a strength. I was not going to let myself be overcome by weaker beings without fighting. On the other hand, there are the fears, the worries, the insecurities. This is what extinguishes the fire. I was an addict, and I had also fears, worries and insecurities. Finally, intelligence directs everything, though it is not always in control. Common sense, however common it may be, must be trained, just as any other skill must. One also has to develop authority. I did not even consider the defense against physical aggression, power. They were many, and I was not trained for that, nor could I even attempt to be. Yet I had not done military service, for I declared myself a conscientious objector. I did not do it because I was afraid of or rejected weapons or the army. In fact, at eighteen, I wanted to do military service in the COES, the Special Forces, but my father convinced me to continue studying. I objected because I had heard so much about hazing, and I was unwilling to tolerate anyone humiliating me in that way. In college, I witnessed the abusive treatment to the rookie students in dorms. I was never going to go through something like that. If my attackers were real people, my intention was to discover them and report them to justice. They were committing a flagrant crime, perhaps even more than one. That was my only aspiration. Until then, I had to neutralize the psychological and emotional effects they had on my mind. As Quilapayún said: "Close the wall!"

There was another most likely option: they were only hallucinations – perception without an object. There is an old philosophical theory, the solipsism of Bishop Berkeley, which more or less says that the world does not really exist except in our minds. God induces everything we perceive in our senses, creating the reality in our mind, as in *The Matrix*. As Descartes – another philosopher – said, we can only be sure of our own existence. Whether or not it has an object, the perception of the voices is there, and, therefore, it is real. It is almost impossible for one's mind to understand it another way. In fact, that would virtually be a pathological symptom, a bit like not believing in the existence of the things one is seeing with one's own eyes. It is understandable to be afraid of real beings, especially if they seem aggressive. I had fear, but hallucinations, whatever they are, cannot do anyone physical harm. They can only speak.

I overcame the fear of physical assault by exposing myself to it. I was following the principle of parsimony, Ockham's razor: the simplest, and therefore most likely, was that they were hallucinations. They couldn't harm me if I went about my usual life, only if I stopped doing that. Then they would do me serious harm without even touching me. Feeling afraid is like feeling any other sensation. It's not pleasant, but it can be borne if one doesn't focus on it and doesn't let it grow. One has to let it pass through the body like a wave, ignoring and not trying to dominate it. One has to be the spike that bends so as not to be broken by the wind. Pain is not pleasant either, but one can have a regular life with it. If one responds to fear or discomfort, anxiety rises, and anxiety feeds them. So I would relax and let fear flow through my guts while trying to cultivate and grow other kinds of emotions that were more useful to me against the voices: rejection and determination. There is no place in the body for so many feelings at once. They compete with each other.

Finally, those emotions displaced fear. Nothing bad ever happened to me. Once I got used to it, things started to lose intensity quickly. The recklessness that drove me to risk my life by consuming high doses of drugs paradoxically helped me in this task of desensitization to fear. If I was not afraid of dying or something worse by poisoning myself, why was I scared of what these entelechies could do against me?

When the fear of physical assault is removed, the real fight against the voices begins. Against oppression, one has to resist, and in this case, the oppression is done through speech. The opposition must also be on the same ground. Power and authority, though they are often exchanged, are two radically opposite concepts. Power allows you to compel others, authority enables you to convince them. Power is pure physics, authority is the highest degree of human development. Power causes rejection in many people. Power can be, and often is, abusive and oppressive. Authority is positively valued, admired, sought. For that reason, the mighty people prefer to be called 'authorities' rather than 'power'.

The voices wanted to have authority over me, but they were only capable of aspiring to power. They would have all the power that I would allow them to have. They couldn't hurt me physically but emotionally. They could also be very annoying. They could distract me when I talked to other people, or try to prevent me from sleeping – and this is very dangerous for one's health. They attempted to exasperate me all the time. Stress is a weakening thing. They took advantage when I was in a slump to use their most aggressive or sarcastic tone, making my situation worse. They were not harmless in that regard. In the long run, they could cause as much damage as a beating, possibly more. Stress causes the body to generate substances that can be toxic, such as the hormone cortisol. The voices can lead the listener to suicide out of desperation.

In my particular case, I decided that what I should never allow, under any circumstances, were the voices to inspire in me even a dab of respect. They were aggressive, oppressive, abusive, bothersome, mean. We have a cultural bias that leads us to misinterpret dominance as authority. There is an old remedy for this that the powerful have always feared, an infallible remedy: mockery, ridicule. In one Schopenhauer's essay, I read that the custom of challenging someone to a duel for honor was abandoned, not because of prohibitions and persecution, but when people began to laugh at the duelists and ridicule them. It is not very honorable to be taken for a clown. The ridiculous does not convey authority, so once I found the ridiculous side of the voices, the rest was a piece of cake.

In that sense, I must admit that I had it easy. I am not an arrogant and conceited person; I think that that is a weakness. Whoever thinks they is at the top no longer climbs higher. But I cannot but affirm that I seemed to be much smarter than all my voices put together. There is a very witty saying: 'The intelligence of a lynch mob is equal to the intelligence of the dumbest one of them divided by the number of members.' I told them that many times, trying to guess who the dumbest one was. Instead of focusing on the hurtful things, I tried to find the ridiculous, absurd, stupid face. I was trying to be objective: I imagined real people doing what the voices did as though I were a beholder. Aside from giving them ridiculous nicknames, I criticized their methods and tried to come up with better ones, as if giving them lessons. I didn't forgive any nonsense from them; all of their bullshit was motive for derision. I have never laughed more at something than at my voices.

It is said that laughing is very healthy, and my laugh was sincere, the healthiest laugh of all. Laughing lifts the spirits, strengthens the soul, increases self-confidence. It is clearly preferable to negative feelings – anger, resentment, bitterness, fear. But the voices also defended themselves. Sometimes it went wrong and backfired. If I messed up and they managed to embarrass me, their counter-attack began. Then it was I who would end up emotionally beaten. It was an all-out struggle, but it was also training. The bad blood of the voices seemed to increase, and that empowered me. I often said to them: "Remember that it is you who want something from me, not me who wants something from you." 'Who pays the piper calls the tune.' And, honestly, I didn't want anything from them. I wasn't going to allow them to have something to negotiate with. The goal was not to get them to shut up but to take away all possible value from their words or feelings. I had to utterly despise, ignore, obliterate them. Whoever lives by the sword dies by the sword.

Regarding the supposed human counterpart of the voices – the people I believed existed behind them – I was also trying to put some plans into practice. In the beginning, when I thought they were normal, ordinary neighbors, I tried to annoy them back using a cassette tape with a recording of insufferable squeaks. The tape had the form of a Moebius band, an infinite loop. These tapes never ended, so I left them playing at the window one morning when I went to work. Throughout the day, I regretted it. It would be bothering people who had nothing to do with the situation. When I returned home, I had only one thing on my mind: turning off the damn tape. I think it bothered me more than anyone else. I did not repeat it.

I remember a particularly surreal scene: I am in my living room, eating a plate of lentils. In the chair beside me, the tiny Mus is on a cushion looking at me with pleading eyes. 'Why have you left me over here? I want to be on your lap', he seems to tell me. The blinds are lowered to make it difficult to see inside, but Gasparín and his minions lurk outside. They can see through the slats; they have devices. Behind us, facing the window, is a 1500 watt halogen spotlight. The heat is stifling, but the protests from the unrepentant peepers make up for it. Fuck them all! I greedily swallow the food as large tears roll down my cheeks. I feel entirely distressed, not so much by the pressure of the spies as by the poor Mus, whose eyes beg for me to take him in my arms. Between mouthfuls, I sniff a bit of crushed pill that I keep in a small jar. They were difficult times.

Sometimes, when I was alone at home, to silence the never-ending chatter of the voices, I hummed a kind of improvised chant the lyrics of which were a series of ways to call the voices in general stupid, or to call stupid whoever was speaking at that particular moment. After a while, I would end up hearing a howl like a whiplash, something like "SHUUUUUUT UP NOW!" from one of the voices, usually Gasparín. And I would shut up, having accomplished my goal.

In the beginning, I also tried to use a rapprochement-oriented approach to lighten the mood and end the war. I invited the voices to play with a video game at home, as I had done with Taxi Driver & Sons. They always refused. I tried to negotiate with Gasparín, but he was adamant. The issue was no joke to him. I also invited them to meet in a bar to discuss the matter as civilized people, on neutral ground, and before witnesses, but no way. I even encouraged them to report me to the police, hoping I could at least get to see their faces in a court. Naturally, none of these offerings were taken up.

Since I couldn't spend the day quarreling with them, I used music to do it for me. I like hearing music all day, all kinds of music. There are songs for everything. Many of the lyrics are critical. They can give someone a dressing down. Even if one can't speak, one can communicate pretty well with others using the appropriate song, like in a musical. I have always played a lot of music. Since it was the time when everybody could fraudulently download any song or movie from the Internet, I had more than enough - thousands of songs. And if I needed any more, I would look, find, and add it to the repertoire. There were many songs appropriate for each character and situation. I especially remember the album *¿Dónde Jugarán las Niñas?* (Where Will the Girls Play?) by the Mexican group Molotov. In the office, my workmates also played music all day. They loved this CD. The different songs gave me ideas about the voices. At home, I put that CD on a lot. Some themes became iconic: '*Mátate teté*' (Kill yourself), '*Chinga tu madre*' (Fuck your mother), '*Puto*' or '*¿Por qué no te haces para allá... al más allá?*' (Why don't you go there... to the afterlife?).

I was not sure whether the voices were bothered by the songs, but it helped me. In addition to having fun listening to songs that I liked, I had a kind of automated system that did the dirty work. It was like a robotic personal assistant. I amused myself looking for songs to mess with the voices, and that was the important thing. They were not going to be able to defeat me.

The Nutty Professor

After earning a salary without working for three months, I decided to finally look for a new job and so end that situation, which I considered unnecessary and unjustified. I didn't want to continue writing software as I had developed a kind of phobia towards this activity. I supposed that I could do well as a teacher in an academy with the experience and knowledge that I had accumulated. I got on with it. I had managed to stop taking pills, gradually reducing the daily amount. The voices, however, seemed in no hurry to disappear. They were still in the trenches, as hell-bent on their sickly harassment as ever.

It didn't take long for me to find an ad requesting a teacher for a well-known academy. I showed up for the interview, and the truth is that it was straightforward, as I had no problems getting them to hire me. It was a course on networks, a subject in which I had theoretical and practical knowledge. I didn't have much experience as I had only been helping to assemble and set up the network in my previous job and my own at home, as well. It wasn't my speciality, but I could try it.

It was one of the courses offered by the INEM (National Employment Institute) to help retrain unemployed people. The academy was a private center, so I suppose they received a hefty grant for teaching these courses. They must have had a fixed date to start, and they wouldn't have found a qualified teacher, so chances were they had to settle with me. I had to start that same afternoon. It was a fluky coincidence that saved them at the last minute.

They were a stressful three months, in which I discovered that I was not suitable for teaching the course. The students were totally unmotivated and the heat of the summer afternoons turned the five long hours a day of class into a kind of meeting of narcolepsy patients. The only one who didn't fall asleep was me. We even set up a network, but that didn't work either. The only thing I achieved was that, instead of falling asleep, the students spent all their time surfing the Internet. The voices did not bother me during the course; they were still there, but they seemed to give me a truce. I was working; apparently, they cared about that a lot.

Woefully, during the course, a troublesome event happened. On the way from the subway entrance to the school, they were two pharmacies. The academy was in the Vallecas neighborhood, and that was unexplored and virgin territory for me. I used to wonder as I passed by, with unhealthy curiosity and itchy fingers, whether the pharmacies in this district would be fruitful in terms of getting my inadvisable drugs. Curiosity killed the cat, and one fateful day I decided to try my luck: 'Just a little box.' And so that was how I went back to consuming d-MPH.

Lucy in the Sky with Diamonds

After finishing my painful experience as a teacher, August arrived, and with it, Bonita's holidays, so she and I went on a trip to a campsite. It is cheaper than a hotel, and it is easier to meet people there. We wanted a varied holiday, to find places where we could have a good time. That year, we planned to go for a week to Blanes, on the Costa Brava, and then another week to Sitges, near Barcelona, at my sister's suggestion. She had recently been there and recommended it to us because of the beauty of the place and its everlasting party nights. Mi Niña's brother and his girlfriend stayed in our apartment looking after the cats.

'They' were also on the train on which we travelled to reach our destination. There might have been two or three henchmen, but none of the honchos. They were somehow unconcerned about us, it was mere routine. I was trying to figure out who they could be, but every time I looked back, I didn't see anyone suspicious. They spent the entire trip whispering and talking about me. If we went to the cafeteria, they always followed us at a distance. It was impossible to see them when I looked directly at the point from where the conversations seemed to come. However, there was no doubt that they were there, lurking, watching.

We arrived in Blanes and located the campsite. Nothing remarkable happened there, except perhaps the mandatory visit to the Marimurtra Botanical Garden. The atmosphere was very familiar. The party zone seemed dedicated exclusively to the '*guiris*'. The second day, a family pitched a huge tent, almost a house, next to us. The campsite manager asked us to move to a tiny corner so that the family that occupied the big tent could park their car. The voices had also been installed in the campsite, somewhere. They continued with their constant chatter. What professionalism those policemen had! Anyone would say that they were there more by coercion than for anything else; maybe at the whim of their superiors, and that's why they acted as if they couldn't care less and without any interest.

The fact is that it was oppressive to have them behind me all the time, even when they showed that listless attitude. Another person's attention on us, in turn, forces us to pay attention to them. It makes us spend mental resources, energy. It is an intrusion into our space. My patience was being tested in extreme conditions. I had no choice but to try and have a nonchalant attitude too. Otherwise, it would seem as if I was trying to avoid the world. One cannot pay full attention to two or more people speaking at the same time. Mi Niña got cross when she talked to me and realized that my attention was elsewhere, so I had a double problem. She said that I turned my eyes 'inward', and that it was as though I had suddenly left for another distant place.

Given the situation, a couple of days ahead of schedule, we left Blanes and headed to our second destination: Sitges. The image of the place I had in my mind was quite idealized. My sister had compared it to Ibiza, which I didn't know either, but of whose mythical parties I had heard tell wonders. Besides, Sitges is a major gay tourist destination. At that time, I considered the gay scene as a perpetual carnival in ordinary conditions. On holiday it would have to be something unspeakable. I guessed we were entering a completely different world from the one we knew. For me, Sitges was one universe where anything could happen, where everything was allowed.

As it seemed that the occasion might warrant it, I had brought a couple of acids that I kept in the freezer, just in case the moment arose. They were left over from an outing to the countryside with friends a couple of years ago. An acid is a small piece of blotting paper with an LSD drop, a potent hallucinogenic drug. I should have been afraid to take such a powerful hallucinogen while being besieged by all those phantasmagoric entities, shouldn't I? Well, I wasn't. We had not saved any extra money for the holidays so we practically had only enough to eat and pay for the campsite plot. Around us, the place was full of people, music, and partying. It is a terrible idea to go on holiday to a village such as Sitges without taking a proper provision of funds. We were drooling. We even searched the ground desperately for some money dropped by a careless tourist, unluckily without success.

We decided to make use of our hallucinogenic resource, which was at least free. When the acid started to take effect, we got overwhelmed by so many crowds. Too many stimuli that produced in us an inadvisable feeling of distress. That foreshadowed a bad trip. We retired to the tranquility of the campsite so that the trip started a little smoother. In the silence and darkness of the night, the situation became more bearable. The voices spoke about it as they had also installed themselves at the campsite but, in my state, I didn't pay any attention to them. I was focused on other rather more stimulating and suggestive stuff. Once we reached the peak, the campsite became too small, and we decided to return to the town, not to its crowded streets, but to the beach, where there was hardly anyone, just some scattered groups of lads drinking or couples of lovers.

The hallucinations produced by the acid were mainly visual, some distortions of the edges of things and colors. The sand seemed to be made of a tangle of writhing octopus tentacles. The waves were like glass; they seemed almost frozen. Also, the interpretation of things was distorted. The jetty's rocks looked magical, with faces of mythological beings and strange signs engraved on them. They gleamed with an iridescent and phantasmal light. The cracks between them were mysterious and unfathomable chasms. The stars were huge and very bright. Occasionally, we would see a meteor crossing the sky. They were so big that they looked like the star of Bethlehem. But I perceived all this being aware of where it came from. It didn't give me a feeling of realism, like auditory hallucinations. It was like wearing virtual-reality glasses. Also, running through my body, there were strange physical sensations, and illuminist thoughts, of the kind where one finally understands the meaning of everything, which could only be experienced under a mental state like that.

On the seafront, there was a traveling exhibition: 'At Full Speed'. It warned anyone who wanted to hear about the dangers of designer drugs. There were numerous photos of different types of colored pills. The posters were large so that one could quickly learn how to recognize them. A series of screens featured infomercials on the subject. A little further down, on the beach, there was a chemical toilet, a privy. I wanted to piss, and there we went. Upon entering, I was hit with an intense strawberry chewing-gum smell. It was the smell of the disinfectant, but I'd never smelled it before and didn't associate it with that. I saw the crapper as a mouth full of teeth. The teeth were blunt, not sharp – one had to be able to sit down, didn't one? It was like the Rolling Stones mouth, but without the tongue. Undoubtedly, it would come out later, when one had finished, to clean the bum. *Well, this is Sitges, it is normal that even the toilets on the beach are extravagant*, I thought as an explanation.

When I was about to pee, I saw a lever at my side, with a sign that begged me to pull it when finished. Then I understood everything: when one pulled the lever, a giant ball of chewing gum would inflate from inside the toilet, exploding and leaving the poor user covered in dirt. Only someone who was spaced out would use a toilet like that. It was all a trap from the seafront exhibition. Surely, there had to be a camera somewhere. Then the image might appear on one of its screens with the caption: 'This is where you end up if you take drugs.' I got out of there in a hurry. "I'm not going to pee here," I said with suspicion to Bonita. She used the privy instead without seeing anything unusual. We looked for another less ominous toilet somewhere else on the beach. Luckily, there were several.

We spent the night wandering the beaches from end to end and back again. Everything felt very calm and civilized, as if we were in an exhibition or in a museum and we commented on everything we saw and felt. We carried a bottle of water that we steadily refilled in the footbaths on the back walls of the beach. Occasionally, we would sit on the seafront, with our feet dangling over the sand. I heard my chasers passing behind us. They were with other local civil guards, who had come from a supposed barracks that – I don't know where I got this from – was located further up the street. They were not on duty, but going off partying. When they passed, they made comments about our state: "It doesn't matter, they are drinking water," they said, making little of it, and passed by. I wasn't that interested in paying attention to them at the time. I had better things to look at. I didn't feel threatened by anything at all.

Nothing more remarkable happened in the long hours in which the drug took effect. Shortly before dawn, we returned to the campsite. I remember that, before going to sleep, I thought something like: *I wish that tomorrow when I wake up, the whole thing will have disappeared as if it has all been a dream*. I meant the voices, of course. And the fact is that when I woke up the next day, I noticed a dead silence. There was the traffic noise, the peculiar cooing of turtledoves, the sounds of pots, and people talking. Real people, the kind you can see when they talk. But there were no voices.

I thought it might be a ploy, that they would suddenly appear again to throw cold water on my enthusiasm, as punishment for my excesses the previous night. I tried to concentrate, but couldn't hear anything at all. My wishes had been fulfilled. I did not hear them again during the days I was in Sitges. There were no more highs, for we had no money. Just a few tablets from my recently resumed vice and a couple of joints of marijuana leaves. We went on long walks through the streets, scrutinizing every corner looking for lost money with which we could have a drink in one of the ubiquitous tempting-looking pubs. We never found a penny, so we left there with a promise to save money and return next year. We swore to return with as much as possible. We had to taste that inviting environment.

After that, we still had a few days with my parents and my brothers to the north, to Cantabria, in a peaceful little village near San Vicente de la Barquera. The voices were still not there. I thought I was finally rid of them forever. Sadly, upon returning to Madrid, things changed again. Little by little, in a matter of days, the voices reappeared as soon as the relaxation of the holidays ceased. It wasn't going to be that easy to get rid of them.

Business as Usual

The voices that reappeared after the holidays were the same characters as before. Nothing had changed. Since I believed I was mixing hallucinations with real people, the explanation for their disappearance and reappearance was that only the hallucinations had gone. Real people, like Gasparín, had never left Madrid. I was out of work again, and again I spent most of the day at home alone. The surveillance resumed. Gasparín and his friends began pestering me anew, without stopping. I suspected that they were using my hallucinations against me, taking advantage of the situation.

They were all resolved on getting the municipal police to break into my house finally to search it, and they soon got in the habit of frequently ringing them. The scene was always the same: the police came and the voices released an endless litany of accusations about my numerous sins and offenses. In response, the officers warned them to leave me alone, for they were doing something illegal. Then, the cops left, leaving the voices disappointed. I tried to take advantage of these continuous visits. I thought about getting messages to the onlookers, to let the authorities – the real ones – know that I was aware of the situation and was sick of it. I couldn't go to the police station or the court to report them without evidence. I had to attempt some other way to end it all with that gang of crazy fanatics, especially with their ringleaders.

So, when I was alone, I would put notes, handwritten in large letters, in places that were clearly visible through the windows, but not from the street. I still have two of them: *I haven't called the police yet, but I will call them if you don't stop spying on me all day, you crazy motherfucker!* And *I'm going to denounce you, asshole! You are boring me, you shitty* voyeur, *I am being too lenient*. It was a rather oppressive situation. I felt spied on all day, baited with derogatory comments and threats, with all sorts of gibes and reproaches. They repeated their mantra, "Change your attitude," over and over.

Gasparín even contacted my landlords: a woman and her husband. She was the owner of the apartment, had several flats, and lived off the rent from them. Every month, she dropped in to collect the rent in cash, giving us the corresponding receipt. I remember a day I had heard Gasparín arguing with her and trying to convince her that I had to be thrown out of the flat. She refused to believe him and said that we always paid the rent on time and that she was not going to do so under any circumstances. He stubbornly insisted. Afterwards, she came to our flat, as she always did. She asked for permission to come into the living room to talk about something that I can't recall. I took it as a kind of test. As though she was evaluating what my arch enemy had been telling her. As if trying to inspect the flat's interior. Then, she left and continued arguing with Gasparín in the street, out of my sight. She wasn't going to ask me to leave and urged him to leave me alone. She owned more apartments in the building and would be talking to other neighbors on the stairs or on the street. Or maybe it was all in my mind. The fact is that everyone could end up appearing in my delusions as a guest artist.

For a few days, funny things happened. The voices called the cops so often that they got fed up. Every night, the situation ended up like a TV comedy: the police arrived. They argued with Gasparín, who frantically urged them to take my apartment by storm. Finally, the officers got angry and arrested Gasparín, amid raging protests. Gasparín left the scene, asking his lawyer to get him out of jail. The rest of the voices stayed, and we all breathed a sigh of relief. They were also a little weary of the situation. Gasparín had them mobilized around the clock. They needed a break. His pressure would continue, but no longer so angrily. It would be calmer.

The first time, I was pleasantly surprised. Timber! Justice had finally been done. I was desperately hoping that the police would contact me to file a complaint. No one ever called. The next day, Gasparín reappeared, as irksome as ever. Although that kind of daily theatrical performance never ceased to be funny, I ended up feeling like it was the voices that were having a new joke on me. Or perhaps it was a kind of gift to give me a few minutes of rest and relaxation at the end of the day, after being beaten. I also thought it was proof that everything was in my head, for it was too ridiculous, but that did not stop me completely out of my delusions. Something in the depths of my mind insisted that if I heard people speaking, there were people. That was not negotiable.

Staying at home wasn't helping much either. I no longer had my job as a teacher. Neither did I want to go back to that unpleasant experience. I also didn't want my former bosses to continue paying me for nothing, so I decided to go back to my previous job. I was welcomed. The company was in a good place. They had got a pretty substantial contract with some major companies to develop an e-learning platform (computer-assisted teaching). There were many tasks to perform. Concentrating on work didn't silence the voices, but it kept me busy, and I didn't mind listening to them. I could even quarrel with them while working. They never managed to spoil my work.

Gasparín also used to come by the office every day, to talk to my boss. They used to spend hours arguing loudly, A, trying to throw him out, and he, endlessly insisting. He was tremendously, obsessively, sickly insistent. The rest of the troops waited outside, talking about me, as usual. They seemed to be stationed in the building opposite. There was a large window of smoked glass that prevented seeing inside, although I supposed that, in all probability, they could see me. These guys were more twisted than Fu Manchu. They wanted to hang me, and they had the means and power.

At the end of that year, I finally decided to stop working as a freelancer. I always had trouble paying off taxes, mostly because of the paperwork. I was also a disaster with VAT; more than once I had to ask for a moratorium. The company hired me as one more employee on the staff. Once again, I made the firm decision to stop taking the damn tablets once and for all. I knew that, if I didn't, I would have severe health problems, and, sooner or later, my work would be affected. Bonita was also overwhelmed by the situation. It was not fair and had to be stopped.

I thought about resorting to some professional help. I didn't have much faith in it, but it was clear that I couldn't trust myself either. We had recently met a psychologist through a friend of Mi Niña, so I made an appointment with her and prepared to start some type of treatment or therapy, to see if that worked.

Therapeutic Wanderings

My psychologist belonged to the cognitive-behavioral school. For me, this therapy was irritating and artificial, although I know that it is nowadays considered to be the most effective in a wide range of cases. I preferred to have long talks about what was going on in my head, trying to discover how to control my behavior through self-knowledge and psychoanalysis – or, which is the same, exhibiting myself before the psychologist. I wanted explanations, I already had methods. This system seemed too mechanical to me. I had to write down the relevant events that triggered stress or the desire to consume drugs, and then find possible strategies to neutralize them.

The psychologist recommended that I do some relaxation exercises several times a day. It was a nuisance for me to have to keep an eye on everything. I had the feeling that I was interfering with my own behavior, with my usual way of thinking, and that everything would be distorted by that interference. Observers modify what they observe. The relaxation exercises did not relax me at all. It was supposed to take months for them to work, but I suspected that they were going to be useless. I felt stupid writing down what I thought. It was as if I was making it up because those thoughts arose from the need to write about them. It was the Ouroboros, the snake devouring its tail. Instead, I drew a graph of the progression of my daily pill consumption, to be aware of the dosage decrease, which I decided upon myself. I am always so technical.

At that time, I also became interested in self-help books. These are like a pile of straw in which it is possible to find some golden needle. Out of the blue, you can find an interesting phrase that becomes a reason for reflection, a fertile seed from which countless profitable ideas emerge. They are phrases like 'know yourself', 'things are how you take them', and others like that. They do not have much meaning, but they point in the right direction: towards a path that can even lead to the foundation of extremely fertile philosophical systems. They are much better than the recipes indicating all the steps to follow mechanically, already chewed and digested. They were extra help, almost the best of all.

When I explained about the hallucinations to the psychologist, she said she had to review some documents on the subject to tell me something about it. In the next session, she explained to me that what I had was schizophrenia. It was a severe mental illness and could not be treated by a psychologist. I needed antipsychotic medication, and she was unauthorized to prescribe it, nor was she prepared to deal with such a case. She recommended I seek psychiatric help. We could continue with the therapy in parallel, or when the symptoms had disappeared by medication. She explained that, in my state, they were not going to lock me up anywhere. I could relax in that sense, the psychiatrists were not interested in locking people up against their will. It would be like going to a doctor like any other.

In a way, I was relieved to be able to quit therapy, as I mainly found it very stressful. Taking medication didn't sound fun, though. I had read about antipsychotic drugs and was afraid of their effects. They also had dangerous side effects. I imagined haloperidol injections, my face swollen and expressionless. I saw myself almost turned into a vegetable. I got goosebumps just thinking about it.

However, I decided to visit the psychiatrist. The psychologist had assured me that they could not force me to take medication if I didn't want to. She also said there were new drugs and that things had been massively improved. I had a picture of a sort of nineteenth-century psychiatry, almost like that from a horror movie. I imagined myself locked up, drugged, trepanned, and electrocuted, mistreated by sinister wardens. It wasn't that bad. My GP referred me to the mental health services of the Community of Madrid, where I explained my case. There, however, they could not treat me until I ceased drug consumption. They didn't tackle that kind of issue. I was referred to a CAD (Drug Addiction Care Center) to detox me from the d-MPH.

These centers had proliferated in the wake of the heroin addiction epidemic of the 1980s and 1990s. CADs are facilities with various departments attending to outpatients. There, one has appointments with a social worker, a doctor, and a psychologist. In my case, they were all women, which was fine. For some reason, for these things, I prefer to be treated by women instead of men. They give me more confidence, and I find it easier to open up.

On a first visit, I explained the case of my toxic consumption. I didn't tell them about the voices, just about the drugs I was taking. These centers specialized in the treatment of heroin addicts. Cocaine, a stimulant too, like d-MPH, was already a big problem in those days, but heroin was the main one. They didn't appear to pay much attention to my biggest problem: the consumption of methylphenidate. They focused mainly on the secondary one: the intake of codeine, an opiate, like heroin. I had been reducing consumption substantially during the time that I had been having therapy with the psychologist. At that time, I was hardly consuming anything. They asked me to stop doing it completely, and so I did.

The doctor, to prevent me relapsing on codeine, prescribed the usual treatment to ensure heroin withdrawal: naltrexone, an opioid antagonist. It is taken daily by mouth and nullifies the effect of these substances if one takes them. One can do it, but it's like drinking water. I insisted that the problem was the stimulants, but there was no antagonist for that, and they gave me nothing. For them, the problem was codeine. Stimulants, unlike opiates, were scarcely addictive. They didn't appear to take psychological addiction into account. Maybe they thought that was just an issue for my therapy with the psychologist. Every time I visited the CAD, I had to urinate in a jar, under the close supervision of a nurse or a former addict, so that I wouldn't do the old switcheroo. This way, they would detect if I had started taking the pills again.

The center was always full of pretty wretched junkies. Usually, one goes to a detox center when one's already desperate, on the verge of destruction, and heroin is highly destructive. My case was an exception; it was out of the ordinary. My stubborn persecutors believed that I was doing the right thing by going to the center, but, even so, they didn't stop bothering me. They continued following me everywhere, watching me relentlessly, commenting on almost everything I would do or say. I remember a day when I was sitting in the CAD lobby, waiting for my turn, doodling in a notebook. The drawings showed Gasparín falling from the rooftops and crashing. I drew with tense strokes, as a kind of relief. I was not exactly relaxed in those days.

The social worker was not very helpful to me. I had the feeling that she was releasing a kind of standard peroration that did not really fit my specific situation: I had to find friends who didn't take drugs, I had to perform outdoor activities, I had to play sports, I had to stay occupied... I spent almost all day with people who didn't take drugs, had a lot of hobbies, and had a stimulating and creative job. I suppose she had never been presented with such a case. It seemed like a waste of time for both of us, but it didn't bother me either. I saw it as a moment for small talk.

The psychologist was friendly, but she wasn't much help either. We spent time chatting non-stop, but mostly only about her. Whatever it was I would tell her, she always found a way of bringing the conversation round to her and her life. Since I didn't have much faith in psychotherapy either, I didn't protest and just chatted with her. The truth is that seeking external help to stop drugs was not filling me with much hope. Well, at least, there were the tests, the surveillance, and the naltrexone. I had to give it time.

The doctor was the one who had it easiest; her role was like that of any other doctor: tests, prescriptions, etc. She appeared to be the most helpful professional, for her work seemed the most productive to me. They had patients in a poor state of health and had to carry out numerous tests to detect the drug addicts' common illnesses and injuries. It was like having a private doctor. I've never had such extensive check-ups before.

The urinalysis trick did not stop me from consuming d-MPH again. Would the doctors detect it in the analyses? Would they only look for opiates? The answers were nope and yep. At least, so it appeared. They didn't tell me anything about it. I decided to quit, without warning, for it was all sounding like a sham to me; I didn't want to give explanations. Without further ado, one day, I stopped going to the CAD. It was like a kind of catharsis, for I also decided to stop the stimulants. I knew I had no choice. Only a firm decision could work. Really, I didn't have too much time left to do it. And the truth is that this time was the definitive one. I never took methylphenidate again – or codeine.

They called home from the CAD and spoke to Mi Niña, alerting her to the fact that I could not just stop the treatment. I would relapse again. I couldn't give her compelling explanations and my credibility was at a minimum. I went back to the CAD, and I explained to them about the hallucinations. I told them a sob story of oppression and torment, only in part true. They couldn't treat that problem, a psychiatrist had to. I was referred, clean and drug-free, back to the mental health service. There were no longer interferences to treatment. This time, they accepted me as a patient. In the meantime, I had developed the hope of being able to get rid of the voices with antipsychotic medication. I also wanted evidence of some kind of brain injury, so that's where I wanted to be.

Medicamentous Odyssey

I thought that getting treatment for psychosis only made sense if I really had psychosis. It was not that I had no reason to suppose it, but I could not avoid doubts. I tried in vain to have the voices prove to me that they were actual people: they could call me on the phone, send me an email, or even an anonymous letter or something. I played the victim as much as I could. I told them that this was already crossing the line, that they could not let me undergo unnecessary treatment with medications that could be dangerous to health.

I had read about the new neuroleptics; they were quite safe, and their side effects were not usually significant. Nevertheless, there was some risk of developing malignant syndromes that could even kill the patient. I tried to appeal to the side of them that believed in the common good. They were forcing a situation in which I was going to have to use public resources for no reason: the psychiatrists' time, the price of medicines, etc. There was no way; they said it was my problem, they were not going to prove anything to me, and it served me right.

My first psychiatrist was a woman. Her diagnosis was that I suffered from toxic psychosis. Since I wasn't quite sure about it, I tried to find out if there was some kind of test that could show if my brain was malfunctioning. It can be done with other organs, I thought, so why not with the brain? At my insistence, she gave me a referral for an electroencephalogram in a hospital. She prescribed me risperidone – an antipsychotic – to begin treatment. I was supposed to start with the minimum dose, 1 mg, but she must have made a mistake when writing the prescription and prescribed a trifold dose.

I bought the medicine at the pharmacy to take it immediately. I was used to using substances to deal with problems so maybe this one would work. I still had some time before going back to work, for it was almost lunchtime, and I lay in bed for a while to wait for it to take effect. The effect of this first dose was somewhat unpleasant. I noticed that my mouth felt dry, and my arms and legs weighed slightly more than usual. The voices didn't even flinch, but I supposed I had to wait weeks to notice any effect on my symptoms. To be honest, I exaggerated the discomfort hugely. I pretended to myself that the voices, which I still believed real people, felt guilty when they saw my discomfort and gave me some clue of their existence. Moreover, I had terrified myself by reading in the leaflet the list of awful side effects that the product could cause. All medicines appear to be terrible poisons if you read their possible side effects. With most of them, you can even die. At the same time, I noticed the error in the dose. I called the office to tell them that I was going to stay in bed, that I wasn't feeling well because they had given me the wrong dose – at the office, they knew all about my problem and my treatment. I stayed in bed that afternoon, trying to convince myself and, above all, the voices that my state was much worse than it really was. The performance was of no use. I called the doctor to inform her of the mistake and to make a new appointment. I did not want to continue taking this medicine. It had to be changed.

Once I decided to undergo treatment, I began to look everywhere for information about psychosis and auditory hallucinations. In my naivety, I hoped that getting scientific knowledge about the nature of the voices would make me see them as a mere symptom, just like psychiatrists did. It was not easy. Almost all the books and websites on the subject were written in English. I had some knowledge of this language, but only of the technical jargon of computing, enough to read, with difficulty, programming books. Most of the writings I found were either brief reports from the patients themselves about their experience with the voices, or academic works with no explanation of the phenomenon of hallucinations. Professionals talked about it as though they were just some kind of pain.

I discovered on the Internet two experts on the subject, Marius Romme and Sandra Escher, who delved into the content and the sense of what the voices said. I could only find one of their books translated into Spanish after a long quest, and it was aimed at therapists. I couldn't find any information that would really clarify anything on the matter. I wanted to know even more than science knows today about the phenomenon. I needed certainties. I wished to obliterate the voices completely. I even considered the possibility of just burning a small area of the brain to achieve it. By then, I had already developed my own strategies to cope with those insufferable parasites. The advice I found did not bring me any new ideas. I felt that I was in a world in which my problem, although quite widespread, was almost unknown even to the few who delved deeper into it. And the rest were not interested in the least.

Also, I had read that antipsychotics worked well against the negative symptoms, but they were of little or no effect at all against the positive ones, especially against hallucinations. Hallucinations were not exclusively associated with schizophrenia. They were reported in other types of disorders, such as depression. Having stopped taking d-MPH and codeine, though not weed, my mood was not very happy. I was physically tired and dejected, and the voices did not help. My sleep pattern was also affected; I slept little and poorly. I was gradually gaining weight and looking much healthier, though the recovery process was slow. The voices continued as usual.

I spoke to the doctor and explained to her that I believed I was suffering from depression. I wanted to change medication as I had not liked the experience at all. After listening to the detailed account of all my symptoms and moods, she proposed a compromise. She prescribed a combination of an antipsychotic and an antidepressant: perphenazine and amitriptyline. It produced in me no adverse effects, so I set out to wait for the outcome. I took it for a few months without any results.

Meanwhile, the day of the EEG appointment arrived. I went to the neurology department at the hospital to have the test, hoping that something strange would be found in my brain. I couldn't understand why I'd had to visit a psychiatrist instead of a neurologist. Based on empirical evidence, they could discover what was damaged in my brain, if there was anything. Only then, could proper treatment proceed, as with any other disease. I used to think of a psychiatrist as a kind of psychologist prescribing pills, but it turned out that they didn't even delve into one's mind. How could they prescribe something for me if they didn't do any tests to find out what was happening to me? They only listened to what I told them, and I thought that some of their patients would give them unreliable information. Their treatments seemed to be based on opinion and not on the scientific method. The EEG was normal. When I explained my case to the nurse, she was surprised by the medication that the doctor prescribed. She agreed with me that maybe I should visit a neurologist. I proposed it in the psychiatry unit, but they ignored me.

All the psychiatrists who treated me from then assured me that there were no medical tests for what was happening to me. It is funny because, at the same time, they consider mental disorders as something with a biological origin. I kept trying to get some more radiodiagnosis tests, but nothing unusual ever appeared. My brain, apparently, worked fine.

The medication did not seem to bear fruit in any respect, either as an antidepressant or as an antipsychotic. The voices were as annoying and aggressive as ever, and my mood ranged from mild apathy to slight euphoria. There came a time when I decided to ask to change my medication again. I was not going to go to the psychiatrist and medicate if I had to continue doing all the work against the voices myself, which was the only thing that really mattered to me. I was there to have my voices taken away, that was all.

I had heard rave reviews about fluoxetine, which works by keeping high neurotransmitter serotonin levels in the neural connections. It prevents its reuptake, once it has been poured into the synapse to transmit the nerve impulse. I was becoming an expert in pharmacology and brain biochemistry, for there was plenty of information on these topics, unlike on hallucinations. I spoke to the doctor again and got her to prescribe me this medication just to try something else. I don't know whether it was because of my expectations, but this drug seemed to work. The intensity of the voices faded until they disappeared completely. It had been months since my first visit to the psychiatrist's office and began taking medication. Finally, I could sigh with relief. I had got rid of the voices (again).

The relief didn't last long as they reappeared after a month. The damn voices adapted themselves to everything I shot at them. They rose from the ashes, like the Phoenix. I persisted for a few more months, encouraged by the initial success of the treatment. Also, fluoxetine did not produce any adverse effects. It was as if I wasn't taking anything whatsoever. But there was no way, they did not leave again.

My confidence in the doctor was under the minimum. I asked to see another doctor, and they agreed. This time, he was a man. He appeared much more efficient than his colleague. The first thing he decided was to go back to antipsychotics. He convinced me that this was what I should take, not antidepressants. He offered to try me on olanzapine. Re its side effects, it could lead to weight gain at worst. With this doctor, I could converse about the content of my voices, although he didn't seem to be too interested in it. But at least he gave me more confidence, so I listened to him and started the new treatment.

I started with a 2.5 mg dose. I had to take one tablet at night before going to bed. That first night I slept long and soundly for the first time in years. The feeling of relief from a proper rest was a great incentive, and I was happy with the treatment just for that. I had tried to sleep using benzodiazepines, the tranquilizers that are often prescribed for sleep problems, but I didn't like the drunken feeling with which I used to wake up the next day. With these pills, I woke up as good as new, as though I hadn't taken anything. I didn't gain weight either. My body tolerated them perfectly. The voices, however, didn't even flinch. This time, instead of changing the medication, the doctor increased the dose until it reached 10 mg, with still no result against the voices. I still take olanzapine today. It has only helped me sleep better, which is important, but it did not fulfill its main objective: to eliminate the voices.

The psychiatrist then suggested trying another new atypical antipsychotic, aripiprazole. He believed that this would work better against hallucinations. I had to gradually withdraw the olanzapine, lowering the dose, while increasing that of aripiprazole. After a few days, when the intake of olanzapine had started to be very little, I found that it was increasingly difficult for me to sleep, and each time I woke up earlier. There came a time when I couldn't sleep at all. I spent several sleepless nights, one after another. I tried some non-prescription sleeping pills, but they only worked for a couple of days. My GP prescribed benzodiazepines, but the result was the same. Finally, I had to give up on the change. I couldn't stop taking olanzapine.

That worried me a lot. I had ended up depending on an antipsychotic to sleep. If I ran out of supply, I would probably die. I tried to quit olanzapine on numerous occasions, gradually reducing the dose. There was no way. I even waited almost a month, not sleeping a single night, until I had to surrender due to a hypertensive crisis. I only managed to lower the dose to a minimum amount, after many attempts over the years. The amount I am taking now is under the minimum dose: a quarter of a 2.5 mg tablet. But I still have to take it. Otherwise, in a few days, I feel palpitations when lying down in bed, and I can't fall asleep. I have been reducing the dose for a year now. I had never managed to lower it so much. This time, I hope to succeed.

My voices are sons of substances. No substance can destroy them, unless it also potentially destroys me. Sudden changes in brain chemistry can make them go away for a while, as well as make them come back. When the organism balances and stabilizes, they always end up reappearing. At no time have they changed their attitude or changed their personality, whatever the substance I'd ingested, legal or illegal. I only managed to do it once, at the beginning of everything, with marijuana, as I already explained, but it seemed more like a hallucination over another one than anything else. It is as if they are actually other people who are not affected by what I take. I can get stoned, but they stay sober. In my case, at least, the solution is not to take alcohol, drugs, or medications. I have to use intelligence.

It Takes One to Know One

A few months after resuming my job, the company moved to a larger office. It was located in the same neighborhood, a couple of blocks away from the old one, very close to the Retiro park. In good weather, I used to walk back home through the park. It was quite a walk, but it was worth it, and, besides, that way I did some exercise; to be sitting all day long is not very healthy. Mi Niña was working at the time on a temporary contract, and some days she didn't have work.

One of those days, I asked her to come to the new office at noon, to see it and meet my colleagues. Sometimes, we would meet for lunch, dinner, or just to get together and have a drink in a bar after work, and she used to join us. Despite the worries and troubles she has had to endure for years, we have always been inseparable. When I do any activity without her, I notice the feeling of being incomplete.

She rang the intercom, but instead of coming up, she asked me to come down, with a tone of concern. I did so and found that she was accompanied by J, an old high school friend of mine whom I had not seen for a long time. He had been part of my clique of close friends in my early youth. It was the eighties. The Madrid scene was in full swing: many bars never closed; there were concerts in the parks, day and night, and in legendary clubs, like the Rock-Ola. In the last two years of high school, we spent more time on the street than in the classroom, since attendance was voluntary. We partied all day and night or drank beer on a bench in the Plaza de Barceló, which was in front of the school.

Besides music and partying, something else was booming in those days: drug abuse. Pharmacies supplied countless medications that could be used as drugs. There were barbiturates or strong opiates in many pain relievers. In slimming pills or cold medicines, there were often also amphetamines. In the eighties, also in vogue, was a cousin of the Horsemen of the Apocalypse: heroin.

Things were running wild, and I ended up separating from my friends because I saw that the track we were on would lead us to the abyss. And so it happened for most of them, who stopped studying or working and centered full-time on drugs. I started relating to more ordinary people, also party animals, but whose parties didn't swallow all their time and resources. My sister got me into the mod craze of that time, centered around the clubs in the Chueca neighborhood. There I would end up meeting Bonita, my life partner.

Occasionally, I would see some of my old friends. They faced prison, rehab centers, homelessness, AIDS, or even death. I used to meet with my friend J to do something as innocent as playing chess and chatting for a while. J had ended up opting for cocaine. Many heroin addicts abandoned horse by replacing it with blow. A different way of finding the wreck. I didn't look forward to seeing them, but I felt uncomfortable rejecting my old friends, as long as they didn't try and get me into their deals.

I was still living with my parents when J would come to my house to play chess. He was having psychiatric treatment. It was evident that he was taking neuroleptics, indeed in high doses, due to his swollen face. Also, he had gained a lot of weight, and he had some difficulty in speaking. But his behavior was not odd in any way. Some time afterwards, when I was already dating Bonita, he invited us to the magnificent house where he lived with his parents and brothers, in the mountains near Madrid. He visited us sometimes too when Bonita and I had moved in together, so he knew my address. We stopped seeing each other for some time, until one day, having already developed my own psychosis, I received a call from him. He told me that another member of the old group of friends had died of an overdose. He was crying, completely heartbroken. But there was something else. He started to tell me a story about the two of them: they had been fighting together at the trenches, under the fire of enemy machine guns. The deceased had saved his life, carrying him until he was safe from the bullets. *He's even crazier than me*, I thought, *he is totally hung up in delusions.* He talked and cried non-stop. I don't know how long I was on the phone, wishing for him to hang up at once. Eventually, I made up an excuse and told him we'd talk another day.

I didn't hear from him again until that day, at the door of my office, next to Mi Niña. He had shown up at home, asking for me. Bonita told him to accompany her, for she was going to the office to pick me up. She soon began to realize that something was wrong. J refused to travel by the subway. There were people following him. He was in danger and both had to go on foot and keep their eyes peeled. It wasn't a big deal, because the office was not that far from my apartment, and then we all met. Mi Niña gave me a sideways look to warn that we had a problem. During the hike back home, we had some small talk, nothing out of the ordinary, except a few references to the indeterminate danger he was in. He would explain the whole thing to us at home.

Once there, he told us that we should no longer go outside. They could kill us. He told us a story without rhyme or reason about secret military missions – I dont know where he got them from since he hadn't even done military service. He spoke of a hand grenade that he had covered with his own stomach to save his companions. When we asked him to show us the scars, he pulled up his shirt and there they were. I don't know what he must have done to end up with those marks on his torso. He also told us that his parents were not his real parents, but impostors. His fake father was a mighty and evil person. They wanted to finish him off and steal his heritage. They had locked him in a psychiatric center where, little by little, they were poisoning him, so as not to raise suspicion. He had escaped and needed to hide where they couldn't find him. His fake father's henchmen were looking for him everywhere.

He did not seem rattled at all. He spoke calmly and seemed to feel safe in our company. He fully trusted us, which was a big problem: we were his only chance. We smoked a joint of marijuana leaves and had a beer. He seemed to relax more, as though he was going back to the good old days at the beginning of our wanderings. I played a CD of Burning, a band that he idolized, and he relaxed even more. While he chatted with Bonita in the living room, I said that I had to call work to explain that I couldn't come back that afternoon, and I went to the kitchen to speak from the extension phone we had in there. I called the office and explained to my boss. Luckily, they were already used to my bizarre behaviour. By the way, I took the opportunity to call J's parents and find out what was really going on.

They told me that he had been admitted to a psychiatric center due to an outbreak he had one night, watching his mother preparing dinner. He thought she was poisoning the food and ran in terror onto the highway near his house. The whole family had run after him to avoid him being hit by a car. In his room, hidden by some books, they discovered a pile of tablets. He had not been taking his medication for months. Also, he had started using cocaine again. That morning he had escaped from the hospital, and they were all very concerned about his whereabouts. I reassured them and told them what had happened. I explained that he was in our home and that he seemed to be in perfect physical and mental condition, in a manner of speaking. They told me that the hospital doctors would call me to give me instructions.

After a while, they called me from the hospital. J begged me not to answer the phone, for 'they' could locate us. We shouldn't have any contact with the outside world. I reassured him that I had to answer the phone because I was expecting important calls. If it was someone unknown, I would hang up right away. I had to lock myself in the bathroom as best I could, stretching the telephone cord, so that I could speak to the doctors without him noticing. Meanwhile, Mi Niña continued chatting with him in the living room, to distract him. The doctor explained that J suffered from strong paranoid delusions, that he needed to take his medication, and that she was going to send some paramedics to my home to take him away by force.

I felt that that would be a kind of treachery. Imagining the scene overwhelmed me. I flatly refused even to give the doctor my address. I told her we would think of something to do and keep in touch. The medication didn't appear to be too important an issue. In fact, it didn't seem to be very useful. We all worked together to come up with a plan to get out of the situation, where he was trying to find a way to escape, and we, a way to return him to his confinement peacefully.

He couldn't stay at home, we made that clear from the beginning. His pursuers would end up locating him anyway, and we had to go out to work. It was only a matter of time. After many brainstorming sessions, we managed to find a plan that seemed acceptable to him, although we had to apply a lot of persuasion. It was almost impossible to convince him to do anything as everything for him was fraught with deadly dangers. The plan was to gather evidence against his father. The mercenary doctors of the evil impostor kept him locked up with a false diagnosis of schizophrenia. We had to go to another hospital and get a diagnosis from other psychiatrists who could disprove the false diagnosis in court. There was no other way out. His captor could not have bribed the entire country; nobody is that powerful.

The next step was complicated. We intended to take J to a hospital where he did not feel threatened. Then, he would be admitted there and transferred to the other hospital. We chose the Hospital Clínico, for it was a large center that gave him certain guarantees of being free from the influences of his chasers. We couldn't simply drop him there, so I contacted them to ask how we should proceed. I was told that a doctor had to visit my friend to write an admission flyer, and then we had to ask for an ambulance to take him to the hospital. Given the exceptional nature of the situation, I managed to get a doctor to come to our home.

The waiting felt eternal to us. We suspected that, if J had time to give the matter some thought, he would find a way to reject the plan, and we would have to start the whole thing over again. I had some advantage for I could understand his mental state; I knew from my own experience how a paranoid's mind works. We distracted him as best we could, looking for conversation topics unrelated to the matter. For his part, he seemed obsessed with knowing the date. "What day is it today?" he asked over and over again.

The doctor finally appeared, accompanied by the police. "It is a matter of protocol," the officers explained to me. As J was a mental patient, they had to accompany the doctor for safety. J flatly refused to let the police enter the house. The doctor managed to convince her escort to wait outside on the landing, and they agreed as long as the door was not completely closed. Next, she set about interviewing my friend. Her first question was: "What day is it today?" to which J answered very proudly with the correct date. He knew every trick in the book.

As he was calm when the doctor saw him, she preferred not to give him any medication without talking to his usual psychiatrists. She gave us a flyer to request an ambulance – more endless waiting; more distraction techniques to stop the plan falling apart. Meanwhile, it was getting dark. We decided that we would also call for a taxi, since we had to accompany him to the hospital as witnesses. Once both vehicles arrived, the moment of truth came; the last step of the plan. As we were about to go down, J refused. All the fear seemed to hit him suddenly. He wouldn't get into the ambulance but he would go in the taxi. "Enough is enough! You are going to get into that ambulance, and we are going to proceed as planned!" I exploded. His attitude suddenly changed to one of total submission, and he meekly agreed. He virtually stood to attention. I managed to go in the ambulance with J to reassure him on the way. The vehicle was a kind of van with a chair to which a person could be tied. There was nothing else. Since we weren't going to go too fast, I would sit on the floor and he in the chair. There was no mention of tying him up, of course. Mi Niña would go behind us in the taxi.

The trip was quite bumpy. J kept approaching the door and practicing a series of movements, as though he was going to open it and jump out. I was praying, already quite annoyed, begging that the door could not be opened from the inside, but I said nothing. We didn't talk much during the ride. I was tired of the situation by then; it was exhausting. I looked through the small window at the back and discovered with horror that we were not heading to the Hospital Clínico. We were going straight to the place from which my friend had escaped that morning. How the hell was I going to get him in there? The paramedics had asked Bonita, before leaving, where they should go, and she had indicated that hospital, as she explained later. It seemed that the problems would never end.

Finally, we arrived at our destination after an endless journey due to traffic jams, for it was rush hour. The paramedics dropped us off in the hospital parking lot and left – their job wasn't to escort us. To my surprise, J calmly entered the building with me. I didn't understand anything, but, to myself, I thanked heaven for the inconsistencies of madness. I found the reception and went in to explain the situation while J waited outside the room. They told me to pass through to the adjacent waiting room until someone came to pick us up. "We are not just ordinary visitors. Is no one going to sort out this issue once and for all?" I wondered with irritation, fearing that everything would be ruined at the last moment when we were almost there. There were quite a few people in the room. J seemed to have complete confidence in what I was doing, leaving his fate entirely in my hands. And I felt like a vile traitor. We had a typical waiting-room chat.

After another everlasting interval, a paramedic appeared with two security guards and asked us to follow them. I couldn't see Bonita anywhere. They led us, escorted and in silence, along a lengthy passage, to the psychiatry section. We went through one security door, which seemed to open to the admitted patients' rooms, and a doctor told me that I could not enter and that I had to wait outside. "Wow, I thought that he was the crazy one!" I heard one of the security guards say, not without reason. He had an eye, he was an old dog.

There I stayed, sitting on a small bench next to the heavy door. There was no one around me, no one entering or leaving. I was waiting again for everything to sort the hell out so I could finally go home to sleep, wishing Mi Niña would appear somewhere. It seemed that she had vanished. But, at last, she came down the corridor. We caught up with each other and waited patiently for someone to come out and tell us something. The doctor had asked us to please wait to explain what had happened to write it on the record. I felt better with Mi Niña beside me.

Two young psychiatrists, a man and a woman, finally walked out of the security door and invited us to enter an adjoining room. There we sat with them at a desk and explained the case bit by bit. The two of them were weird fellows. They kept glancing sideways, as if suspecting something, and had a somewhat strange attitude when listening to us. We both thought that they could be two patients who had taken doctors' robes and escaped as well. They were amazed at the feat we had just accomplished: nothing less than driving a guy suffering from paranoia into the lion's den, on his own two feet and voluntarily.

Friendship is more powerful than medicine. I know that what I did was the best for J, that only that could be done, and that we did it in the best possible way. But I still remember his heartbreaking screams when the security guards grabbed J to restrain him as I walked out of the door, and I couldn't help but feel like Judas.

As for the voices, the incident was like a kind of victory, a way of showing off to them. They could not hide their surprise at the exploit we had managed. I could even detect a touch of admiration. They, like me, also used stereotypes. I was a crazy drug addict, and, therefore, I had to be stupid and useless. However, I was able to do things that did not fit well into this simplistic scheme. That amused me.

Paradigm Shift

In my unceasing quest for information about my condition, I found Intervoice, the international network of voice-hearers. It is made up of people with any relation to this subject and professionals of psychology and psychiatry. Their strategy is to pay attention to what the voices say and manage the relationship between them and the hearer. The patients themselves become, in turn, therapists. Hearing voices is not a disease, but it can lead to one because of the problems it can cause the hearer.

There were many testimonies from people sharing their experience and their tactics to cope with the problem that I had to translate – with difficulty – from English. It was the best thing I'd found on this subject. They were a help, if only as moral support. But, like the medication, they were insufficient. However, it didn't seem like I had an actual problem seen from the outside. Mi Niña sometimes got mad at me. She thought I was using the voices as an excuse when I suddenly stopped paying attention to her or laughed without apparent reason.

As Sun Tzu advises in *The Art of War*, 'Know your enemy'. I realized something relevant: sometimes, it seemed that the voices could read my mind. I always tried to reject this possibility. I thought about the typical image of the guy with tinfoil covering his head. That would be too much. For me, the voices were people, and quite ordinary, too. I considered common people capable of this kind of behavior, and worse. Telepathy seemed like something from science fiction, something preternatural. As a sci-fi aficionado, I have read many stories of telepaths. Too fanciful. What would be next? Aliens? Spirits?

However, the idea kept running around in my head. I began to see the possibility as appealing after weighing it up for a while. Telepaths could be far away; they didn't have to be around to bust my balls. They could know everything that passed through my mind, also what I was doing, without the need to see me physically. We have no evidence that the human mind possesses such a capacity, although even the CIA appears to have taken it seriously in the past. Perhaps it was a good idea to demonstrate its impossibility from a scientific viewpoint and so weaken my visceral beliefs about its nature.

I recalled an Asterix comic book where he and Obelix visit a druid who works as a psychiatrist. A patient walks past them on all fours. "He thinks he's a warthog," the nurse explains. After a while, the patient comes out walking upright. "The druid has cured him?" Asterix asks. "No, but he has taught him to walk on his hind legs, so it is not noticeable," the nurse replies. Maybe I couldn't change the voices' personality, for they were alien to me, but my beliefs were not. Although visceral, my insights were mine. I perceived them as mine. If I had created some grotesque neighbors, I could also turn them into telepaths. At the same time, I felt like a fool to find myself absorbed in these speculations, but the idea was taking shape.

Summer came again, and again we went back to Sitges on vacation, to the same campsite as the previous year. This time, we had been saving, and we had enough money. Again, some voices followed me during the trip. We arrived at the campsite, pitched the tent, went down to the town, bathed in the sea, had lunch in a restaurant, and went shopping. The voices were prowling around all the time. In the evening, we went out ready to see from the inside the wonderful and lively places we'd waited to visit since last year. I had already completely given up methylphenidate. This time, there was only beer and some energy drinks. We danced, had fun, went back to the campsite, went to bed, and slept. Upon awakening, I was a little hungover, but there were no voices. The exorcism had worked again. However, I knew it would only be a short truce. Anyway, that was something.

The campsite was lively. Almost all the people in the surrounding tents were gay –groups of friends, couples. There was plenty of laughter, and it was a breeze to talk to the neighbors. We made a lot of friends, Spaniards and foreigners. Everyone seemed very happy and eager to party. At night, we used to meet in the nightclubs, already with a few drinks in us, and we would hug and dance happily. It was another world. We met three boys from Valencia with whom we became close friends. The five of us started going out together, to the beach, to have lunch, to dinner, and to party. We always had lunch and dinner outside; the tent was just for sleeping. One of these guys was charming, and he knew everybody in the campsite. Soon we were partying all the time, inside and outside the campsite, meeting with other people around someone's tent, drinking, chatting, and laughing. It was an unforgettable holiday. We cried on the train as we left, and swore to return the following year.

In the down time, I kept toying with the idea of telepathy, and it seemed to be getting more and more suitable. I decided to put it into practice as soon as the voices reappeared when we were back in Madrid. I would try to accept that explanation and then refute it somehow. Thinking about it again, it was far less absurd than the belief I had presently: a series of slapstick comedy characters harassing and following me everywhere, impossible to locate or discard. I had to shift the paradigm. If something doesn't work, try something else.

Fourth Time Lucky: Thou Shalt Never Get Rid of Us

On the Sands of Hesitation

The fifteen days of holiday soon ended, and we went back home. It didn't take long for the voices to reappear. I was careful to speak to them only in my head, paying attention to not moving my lips. This way, they could only interact with me if they knew the content of my thoughts. I still had the feeling that they were people in the surrounding area, that they could see me. The voices reacted as if they had been waiting for me to finally understand the real low-down, congratulating me on my discovery. They told me that it was about time I realized what was happening.

Feeling one hundred per cent immersed in a telepathic experience took some time. I was still hesitant, but it became clear that the voices could see not only my actions but also read my thoughts. Little by little, I lost the ability to locate them in the vicinity. The voices ended up suspended at some undetermined point in the sky, far away. Sometimes to the right, sometimes to the left, in front, behind, but always up. I began to explore this new reality and to realize the implications of this new situation.

The worst of it was that now there was no escape. As telepaths, they could scrutinize the depths of my mind. I had nowhere to hide; I was an open book for my stalkers. They would know everything I thought, see everything I saw, maybe even feel everything I felt, though the latter was never clear. They were still people, of course, but I didn't know where they were or if they were together. The characters didn't change, though the police farce had ended. A couple of them were still cops, it was their real job, maybe some of them were also real soldiers, but the important thing was that they were all telepaths. I had made their bullying and wrecking work even easier.

It was time to watch what I thought, too. If information is power, now they had in their hands all the power that knowing everything about me could provide them. Initially, there was a kind of impasse. The voices seemed to be adapting to the new situation, restructuring their strategies, perhaps giving me some time to reflect on my new situation. Maybe they thought that I would become aware of my helplessness and become more reasonable and submissive.

There was a point on which I was always uncompromising. I still demanded a demonstration. I was not going to discuss the matter with anyone without convincing and unquestionable proof of their existence. I had the hand of questioning the reality of the situation as an escape route in tough times, and I was not going to lose it. It was trivial; a phone call, a letter, an email... It wasn't too much to ask.

Back then, the phones did not indicate the number of the caller. They could also use a phone booth. Another option was to create an email account just for the occasion. If they were afraid of being tracked and located, they could take advantage of a trip and do it from a phone box. I tried to give them all possible options so that they had no choice but to do it, no excuse to refuse. I asked them if they were afraid to come out into the open; if they feared that people would reject them, even lynch them. But they were not going to give me any information, not even if they knew one another in person. In their telepathic world, they were governed by their own strict rules: no personal contacts, no one outside it could know of its existence. It was, as they called it, 'the best-kept secret ever'.

Now that I was also one of them, I had to belong willy-nilly to their strange group and to submit to their particular laws. I had no choice. The situation did not seem to have improved in this regard. They were the law, and it was an unquestionable law. The voices I was hearing were like delegates, representatives, a kind of shock group charged with forcing the new acquisitions to integrate into their community. They could not tell me much, everything was top secret there, but they were not alone, there were many more listening to everything we said. There were also children, so we had to be very careful with our behavior, with what we thought. It could cause problems in their development, induce them to misbehave. They had leaders, mighty bosses. I wasn't going to like it if I had to deal with their bosses. It was going to be even worse than with them. The story of the boy who cried wolf teaches us about the problems that arise from deceiving people and teasing them. Finally, nobody believes anything that is said, especially if it is something out of the ordinary. The voices always talked about teasing me, so their credibility was less than zero. I expected to hear a burst of loud laughter just for taking into consideration anything they could tell me. This was already beginning to be too incredible a story. Besides, I was conditioned to make fun of everything they told me. Because of their behavior, I used to say to them that they were more like apes than people. I compared them to *Planet of the Apes*: monkeys capturing humans. That didn't exactly help me to make friends.

To me, this pretense of putting myself in their hands to join a kind of insane sect of mutants, taken from a cheap B movie, seemed absurd and, above all, without being able to allege anything. "You have to do everything we tell you," they used to say. "Well, first tell me what I'm going to have to do, and I'll tell you if I'm willing to do it," —I always replied. That wasn't an option. I had to commit before I knew. Even that was secret. It seemed silly to me. I could tell them I was committed and later tell them to get the fuck out. But no, they would know – the advantages of telepathy. I could only be honest if I accepted it. I could never lie to or deceive them, although they could do it to me. They tempted me with the possibilities: "Wouldn't you rather be like us; be able to hide the thoughts you don't want us to hear or talk to us only when you have something to say?"

Thereby, the period of adaptation to the new beliefs spun around this subject. Of course, we didn't spend all day bargaining, only in the rare moments when they weren't trying to pester me. Bothering was their way of pressure, to force me to do what they considered my duty to them, to have something valuable to put on the negotiating table, even if it was a perverse value. Now, they had fertile ground; they could now freely comment on my thoughts and make fun of them. They could ridicule my attempts to not think about something I felt was embarrassing. For my part, I began to notice and reflect on their suspicious secrecy regarding normal humans – the people who do not possess the 'gift' of telepathy. That seemed like a weak point. Whoever hides does it for some reason.

One More Voice

The most striking thing about the new situation was that I also became a voice for the voices. I appeared in the telepaths' mind as they had appeared in mine. Of course, my case was unique. Perhaps they had been born telepaths, although that was also secret. I had become a telepath because of drug abuse. They knew how to hide their thoughts, just as they knew how to transmit them. However, I was like a kind of radio station that kept broadcasting mine all day and all night. It bothered them, and they wanted me to shut up once and for all. I had to learn to control the phenomenon. They considered me a kind of invader and accused me of being the culprit for everything because of the way I had ended up with the darn faculty.

Their community was purely telepathic. As people, they lived regular lives. There were no gatherings in dark caves to celebrate obscure rituals dressed in mysterious garments. On the airwaves, to put it somehow, they didn't know one another in person; no one knew who anyone else was. Apparently, they used to talk about stuff, though I was never able to find out what the hell they were saying to each other, for the only topic in their conversation was me. They also gave me no clues. In fact, it was impossible to talk to them about anything sensible.

Their inevitable favourite catchphrase always came up right away: "That's none of your business!" Nothing was my business. Anything that could reveal information about them was top secret. I used to end up pissed off and sending them to hell. Then, they would also fly off the handle, the armistice would end, and the pressure resumed. "Since you are not capable of behaving like normal people, behave like savages, which is what you really are," I would say to pique them even more. This, moreover, constituted an escape valve when I felt cornered by their specious malarkey about my obligations to them. "As long as you refuse to show me that you are real people, I'm not going to follow any kind of instructions, no matter how harmless or naive they might seem" – That was always my final answer.

Their particular laws prohibited any demonstration. None of them had ever made contact in – as we called it – 'the real world'. They didn't even use names, since they could address who they wanted, and only them, at will, I surmised, by using some other mysterious sense, although they didn't explain anything about that, either. However, with me, they could make exceptions. They stopped calling me the drug addict and addressed me by my first name: Miguel. Sometimes, I heard them talking among themselves, there in the distance, but I couldn't understand a word. Out of habit, I used to listen to them to try and understand their chatter. They answered in an angry voice that I should not interfere in their private conversations. Then, the attack would start over.

Everything I thought could be used against me if only to make fun of it. Trying to avoid thinking about something was even worse, as well as impossible. The voices would use everything I exposed to annoy me, attack me at will, to demonstrate how much I needed to undergo their telepathic training; like the protection services that the Mafia 'offers'. Diplomacy was not their thing. And these were the supposed welcoming committee, kind of like ambassadors. How would the rest be? Quite a civilization, isn't it?

Leaving aside the question of whether I deserved mistreatment or not, on account of my horrific sins against morality and good manners, what about the unfortunate people they were martyrizing for no reason? Many people were being sectioned in psychiatric hospitals, medicated almost to catalepsy to endure the attacks of their voices. What had they done to them? Did they lead them to that condition just because 'their thoughts bother us'? To this, they replied that this wasn't because of them, that there were also people with real hallucinations. My case was different, a singularity. They did not care about my health or morals, but they thought that I was unreasonable because of drugs, so they had to force me to stop using them.

Another thing that caught my attention was that every one of them spoke my language. Without any identifiable accent. Weren't there also English, Russian, or German telepaths? They replied that, since I didn't know other languages, only those who spoke Spanish could talk to me. But, were there not Galicians, Andalusians, Catalans, or Latin Americans? Another explanation they gave me was that the thoughts were translated into the listener's language. The fact that the thinking was transmitted as words, even with intonation, also raised some doubts. It didn't seem like the kind of mechanism that nature implements.

Thus began the work of questioning the reality of the phenomenon. I tried to devise experiments on a scientific basis. If there was the transmission of something, there must also be the possibility of interference, even isolation. I used to tease the voices by telling them that I was going to discover the particle that transmits thought. I would call it '*putón*' in their honour (from Latin *puto*, *putas*, *putare*, which means, among other things, 'to think'. In Spanish, it is also the augmentative of '*puto*', a disliked expression similar to '*fucking*' in English.) It bothered them that I did not take the matter seriously. That was one of my best assets; to demonstrate that I didn't feel helpless, far from it.

Being inside an elevator did not seem to affect the transmission as the voices were heard just the same. I went to a deep cave near Madrid. Large masses of rock were useless. Distance didn't seem to be a problem, either. I traveled 600 Kms every summer to Catalonia. I also went to Germany once on holiday, but the voices remained unchanged, even in the plane. How much energy was needed to achieve something like that? I was thinking of taking a trip around the world, looking for a point where the whole earth was between me and the telepaths (I didn't consider outer space). There could be no thicker barrier than that. They told me that it wasn't worth the bother. There were telepaths all over the globe. The most reasonable thing was to doubt their existence, but how could it be shown that something does not exist? The absence of evidence is not evidence of absence.

I tried to tempt the voices with the idea of participating in a quiz show. They would tell me the answers and later, we would share the profits. No way. At this point, they were honest, and, besides, it was too dangerous, for I was not allowed to know their identities in any case. That attitude reassured me, in a way, regarding one of my main concerns: the passwords that I used on the Internet to access my bank accounts and the like. Given this bunch of madmen that could read my mind, trying to bother me all day long, it wasn't a good idea that they knew my passwords. They could empty my current account, buy things in my name, cancel my orders, impersonate my identity, and send abusive emails to my contacts. In short, a whole battery of fuck-ups to complement their mental attacks to lead me inside a straitjacket.

Since, more than once, they threatened to do so, I opted to generate long random passwords on the computer. I wrote them in a file and used them by copy and pasting. Only Bonita would know the bank account password, and only she would use them. I explained to her the new turn of events. I said that, though I could reason that everything was only in my mind, I would however feel more comfortable.

Finally, all these pressures, doubts, and fears gave rise to some concession on my part, though with much reluctance. They would soften the treatment for a while. In exchange, I had to make an effort to assimilate my condition, stop getting nervous, and take it as something natural. They believed that my thoughts would be hidden again, and we could all say our goodbyes to each other forever.

The Rain in Spain Stays Mainly in the Plain

The biggest hindrance to breaking the relationship between me and the voices was, without any doubt, Gasparín. He had ceased playing the role of an authoritarian civil guard and become merely a grouchy man. Gasparín was like a nitroglycerin bottle: any slight touch would make him explode. However, he actively participated in the supposed learning process. It did not seem too sophisticated an idea. The fact that I had my attention focused, almost obsessively, on listening to whatever the voices were saying, was the prime mechanism that caused my thoughts to project into their minds. I didn't understand wherefore, if that was so, and they knew it from the beginning, they had been devoted to catching my attention so obdurately, for so long.

They certainly didn't seem like the best teachers ever, the most appropriate people to teach someone to ignore them. Firstly, they were fixated on forcing the situation, on getting me entirely focused on them. Now, when they had got me to collaborate, it turned out that I had to do the exact opposite to undo it all and return to the initial situation – in which I didn't know of their existence. Was it not to distrust their abilities?

From then, there were periods where the voices were quite peaceful and quiet. To me, it was almost more stressful trying not to think about them. If someone tells you not to think about a white bear, the first thing you think about is a white bear. I was inured to spending most of the time struggling with my voices. It was like a kind of background mental process which could be activated without interfering with my regular activities. Like a routine, a habit. It appeared that these telepaths didn't know what they were doing. It was as if they were trying the first thing that popped into their heads, a simplistic common-sense solution, a truism. There were no arcane instructions or procedures, the fruit of ancient knowledge. But the fact was that they were pretty collaborative. There was nothing lost in trying.

Though it was a relief not to hear the voices as frequently as before, I had a kind of automatic radar that continually searched for them. In hearing the slightest whisper, the defense mechanism would activate releasing something like an adrenaline shot, putting me on alert and ready to repel aggression. Any explosive sound, like a dog's bark, turned into a Gasparín rant. There was tension in the air, a stalemate. But the brawl would erupt sooner or later, as though we all needed to release accumulated tensions. In a sense, it was a liberating experience to hear, all of a sudden, Gasparín's authentic howls, once his patience was exhausted.

Though they told me that we could still chat on occasions, like ordinary people, to get used to relating, it never seemed a good time for them. Talking to them was a sterile act; I couldn't ask them anything and nothing was my business. Why did I need to integrate with telepaths who didn't want to speak about anything? Another thing that made good relationships prickly were the ridiculous names I had given them. I should stop calling them Gasparín, Mr Tantrum, Señor Levamos, and the like. It was disrespectful. That was difficult. For me, those were their names. How could I forget, after using them for so long? How was I going to call them if they didn't want to tell me their names? They didn't even deign to give me false names.

They complained that my mind was pandemonium. I was always thinking about something, pondering, chewing ideas. Talking to myself, even the most trivial matters. They said that it wasn't normal. I have heard some people say that they are often not thinking about anything; they just have a blank mind. I find it incredible that this can be possible. I can't imagine myself thoughtless. It would be like being dead. I am unable to do that. I have never succeeded even when I have tried it. Trying to leave my mind blank doesn't relax me, it exasperates me. If that was the way, I couldn't be the walker. Me pretending to stop thinking was already the height of tyranny. I replied that the reason they were barbarians was because of that, for not thinking about what they were doing.

The total loss of privacy was another reason why the presence of the alleged telepaths was exasperating. They said that it was my fault, my problem. They argued that I had to work harder, that they had no interest in my private life, that, in fact, they wanted to stop knowing about it, that it was my duty to leave them alone. I had to get used to living a normal life always feeling watched, and not exactly by friends. I thought about the relationship with pets, for instance. Some people find it uncomfortable that their dog or cat watches them while they are in the loo. Others do not care in the least that they are right there watching everything they do. That's how I had to see those telepaths. These comparisons hassled them a lot, but they helped me to adapt to the situation without making any concessions.

My patience, like theirs, was gradually wearing thin. At times, I recalled everything I had been through, and then my blood boiled and mentally exploded. The voices also exploded more and more often. Some of them even took advantage of the quiet moments to try and sabotage the project.

Sometimes it seemed that the few of us who participated in those explosions were the only ones who realized that, as if the rest of the telepaths were absent on those occasions. Usually, they found out about the matter later at night, when I was already in bed trying to sleep. They reproached both myself and the other folk responsible for the brawl, for our brainless attitude. Sometimes even Gasparín seemed genuinely sorry and claimed he was trying hard, but he couldn't help but lose patience. The situation did not move forwards. It wasn't improving at all.

It was as annoying to hear them only once in a while as it was listening to them all the time. And almost worse was when the voices spoke in a civilized way rather than when they teased and attacked me. The conflict could not be simply ignored and buried in oblivion. Eventually, I gave up my dubious attempt at telepathic education just a month after starting. It never happened again. I had to fight – *Victoria o muerte*.

Freak Show (Again)

After having had a great time that summer during the holidays in Sitges, I decided to go back to going out at weekends. I got so excited that I became a party animal and I couldn't spend any more Saturday nights at home. Mi Niña and I began to frequent the gay nightclubs in our neighborhood, Chueca. In those clubs, Bonita could speak to or dance with whoever she wanted without worry, because everyone knew what her intentions were. The boys often tried to flirt with me. Once I got used to it, I was amused and flattered.

We made many friends and started to move only within the gay scene. I had not become a complete teetotaler. We drank beer and, as the nights were long, we drank quite a bit. We also drank energy drinks and took ginseng pills or some other natural product containing caffeine to compensate for sleepiness and alcohol. In bodybuilding supplement stores, they sold pills containing ephedra, the plant from which ephedrine is obtained, a 'mild' stimulant, but whose unprescribed sale is nowadays prohibited. I continued smoking the occasional marijuana joint. It could be said that, in those first months, I made a life with some excesses, but they were not outside what could be considered normal.

When I was partying, just like when I was concentrating on work, I kept listening to the voices, but my attention was focused on other matters and, at best, I kicked them out scornfully. However, when I was not concentrated on anything particular, I gave the impression that I had attention problems. It was hard for me to focus on something that wasn't absorbing. At those moments, I used to think obsessively about the voices and how to get rid of them. I retired to my inner world. I needed action to relate to the outside world.

Addicts have a tendency to lie, to hide things. In my case, I had developed a kind of compulsive behavior in this regard. Sometimes I would hide even the most innocent things, like a simple bag of sweets. Instead of feeling overwhelmed and helpless about not being able to hide anything from the voices, I tried to act on the basis of absolute sincerity and transparency. I couldn't dupe or hide anything from the telepaths. Is it possible to behave openly in such a situation? Yes, indeed. If something is embarrassing, one has to either accept it or stop doing it. To accept is not the same as to conform. It is about discarding useless and harmful feelings, such as guilt and shame, and analyze the problem objectively. Perhaps, at this moment, you cannot get rid of it, but if you work on it, in the future, you will. This also came in handy in the real world. I had to learn to have nothing to hide, not to lie, or to have no need to. I admit that it took me quite a while.

I had no qualms about telling people about the voices, for I felt the need to talk about it with someone. I always called them hallucinations, of course. I explained the telepathy stuff as exactly what it was, an unavoidable belief. The idea seemed no more absurd to me than the very concept of auditory hallucination, and my mind preferred it. People were not usually interested in the subject. At best, they were curious, but they never tried to drill into details.

It is said that telling someone that you hear voices is stigmatizing, but I think that stigmatization arises when people see you as a weirdo. If you seem normal to them, nobody cares too much. Or maybe they don't want to know, but, apparently, no one felt awkward when I mentioned it. It was like saying: "I have a headache." Not even my acquaintances appeared to be interested in the least. Sometimes they took it as a complaint, as though I were whining. My intention was never to complain. For me, it was a fascinating phenomenon. Besides, it was part of my life experience. I wanted to share it. I did not feel weak or helpless against the voices. Sometimes I was even bothered by the lack of interest from the people I told. It was as though I didn't matter to them, as though I couldn't tell them something intimate about myself, as if they cared for me only at a superficial level. Over time, I ended up resigning myself to not even mentioning it. Not for fear of rejection, but of indifference. When Bonita asked me how were my voices,

I replied that they were fine, and that's it. I didn't want to talk about it as if it was just a toothache. The voices often tried to distract my attention, just to make Mi Niña mad at me, and they usually succeeded. On many of these occasions, I did not even mention the voices. What for, if I was supposed to be okay? It would only sound like an excuse.

In that stage, the plethora of voices received new recruits. Gasparín was starting to appear less and less. He was being replaced as the main nuisance by a new character: *El Zumbao* (the Pixilated). *El Zumbao* was, and still is, diametrically opposed to Gasparín. He is also grotesquely prickly and exaggerated. His stereotype is that of a misanthrope, or perhaps a beggar, someone in an advanced state of social exclusion. His character is bitter, and his ability to express is quite poor. Everything seems wrong to him, to the point that he becomes so exaggerated that one has no option but to ignore him. I gave him that nickname because he was utterly irrational. He talked and talked, and keeps talking non-stop, saying the same things obsessively, going round in circles. He is engaged in a kind of personal war against me.

Usually, he talks to the other voices, constantly repeating expressions like "He has to have a weak point!" or "Something has to be done!". He seemed to want to assume leadership of the voices against me. I used to tease them saying: "This is the perfect leader for all of you! I don't understand how you can stand him without telling him to get stuffed!" Honestly, it seems that he is more annoying to them than to me, though they don't show it, just in case. I asked them if there were many more like that in their community. At the same time, I was wondering what such a character was doing in my mind. What purpose had I for creating him?

Several groups were formed, some of them with a sort of political trend. The builders disappeared as they were out of place. The older ones formed a group with a conservative orientation, always made out of stereotypes. Others, younger, formed a hotchpotch of different degrees of leftism. Both left- and right-wingers are closer to populism than to serious politics, whatever such a thing could be. There are those whom I call '*Los Garrulos*' (the rube-like boasters), whose ideal of socialization is a sort of military hazing and school bullying. These know little or nothing of politics. There are also '*Los Machotes*' (the he-men), who don't mess around with politics. They have a strong and virile personality. They neither defend nor attack me. They are sure of themselves and seem to rejoice when I am like that, too.

They are the stereotype of classic relationships among men, in which self-confidence prevails over sentimentality. It appears that, for them, messing with me is a weakness. They come from time to time, especially on Saturday afternoons, when I am having a drink in a bar with Mi Niña and friends. I try to ignore them. They get into my thoughts, but they don't do it aggressively. With them, I just keep a non-belligerent distance. There are also a couple of guys who claim to be Falangists (a kind of Spanish fascist group). There is even one who says he is a professional politician, and he protests a lot when I am critical – that is, always – of real political issues.

There is one who is specialized in social reprobation, speaking with great moral superiority in a tone of intense disapproval. I call him *'Tío Vinagre'* (Uncle Vinegar), *'Juan el Agrio'* (Sour Jhon), or 'Rafael Amargo' (Bitter Rafael) – with apologies to the great bailaor. There is another who claims he is in prison. He just threatens to hunt me when he gets out. There are a couple of them who seem to be people with mental disorders too, perhaps to give the affair a touch of reality. Sometimes they complain a lot about what I think, other times they strongly agree with me. Occasionally, they cry saying they can't bear the situation. And I often lose my patience and I am rude even with them, which makes me feel kinda guilty. Finally, there are children or adolescents. Those who are apparently more intelligent do not cause problems; they are good boys. The others, *'Los Niñatos'* (the brats), get cocky and try to mess with me with typical adolescent bravado.

The Poverty of Socialism

I divided people into two clearly defined groups: normal humans and telepaths. I considered myself a member of the first group, despite my new and unwanted ability. If I had any duty, it was not to the telepaths. In fact, I claimed that they also had obligations towards others. Our responsibility was to uncover the whole thing so that science could investigate the phenomenon. I used to say that perhaps the cure for auditory hallucinations could be discovered if we all collaborated with science. I told them that there were enough courts, national and international, to settle the case, and theirs was too barbaric a system. I required the mediation of a neutral judge and a trustworthy institution.

But, if they didn't want to demonstrate their existence to me, were they going to do it to some authority? They didn't even want to hear about being in the limelight. They never said anything clearly. It could be that they didn't want to end up in a laboratory being studied as strange specimens. It could also be that they feared ending up being exterminated either by the ignorant masses or by the mighty fearing their secrets to be uncovered. Sometimes, it turned out that they were already secretly serving the state, and I was going to be in trouble if I didn't submit to their plans. With them, it was almost impossible to be sure of anything. They always gave contradictory, wrong, or no information. I would never know the truth about them if I didn't yield to their pressures and integrate. And, even then, they promised me nothing.

The times I analyzed the matter from a more rational point of view, thinking of it as just a mental disorder, I felt that the voices no longer had any purpose. But they had become chronic, and now there was no way to get rid of them. It was as if they had become autonomous entities, living in my mind, but wholly separated from me. Once, they even stated that they were just that. I had created them, and they had a right to exist. But they demanded some control over the body or, at least, to participate in decision making. And I was not going to allow that.

My preferred belief, in any case, was that of the telepath community. It was a social conflict that was easy to reject using logic and the law as a basis. There were no Freudian connotations or hidden traumas. It was just a political cock-up, populism, 'escraches'. I once said to them that no person was the property of anyone else, even in part. They couldn't behave as though I were some kind of slave, with the duty to obey their demands. They replied: "Of course we are all partly owned by others, this is the basis of society, to subordinate individuality to the group." I then called their beliefs 'socialism'; society above all else. Mine, in contrast, was 'individualism'.

They stubbornly repeated that this was a democracy, so we had to vote in order to decide what to do. I replied that this was the type of 'democracy' with which the last century's communist regimes were disguised, such as the Democratic Republic of Germany. Our liberal democracies are based on the declaration of human rights. Nobody can be forced to belong to a group. Voting must be supervised by reputable institutions. There must be independent courts, as well as the necessary conditions so that minorities are not crushed by the dictatorship of the majority, and vice versa. Their supposed political system was naive and seedy. Their political ideas were like something out of a satirical newsletter. It was like an adolescent commune or the council of elders of some tribe of ancient times. I often used the cliché: 'Socialism equals poverty'. When people are subordinated to the group, both get impoverished. Only if one first fully develops as an individual can one enrich the groups he freely joins. I was getting really interested in politics.

They tried to convince me by pressing upon me supposed eternal and compulsory social rules, not of their particular society, but of the real one, the one in the real world. However, it was they who were hiding from that society, not I. Their obstinate insistence, often aggressive, made it clear that they were only interested in social norms insofar as they supported their ends. Harassed by the pressure, I began to call them monsters, mutant offspring who wanted to take control of humanity. But I told them they were lousy offspring. They didn't seem like those powerful and fearsome beings who populate our fantasy stories about telepaths who want to dominate the world; instead, it was something like imagining Dracula shitting. I sent them to hell telling them to go and claim their alleged rights elsewhere. I was not a representative of mankind. I was only a guy whose duty was not to allow the last frontier of a human being's freedom, the intimacy of his mind, to be conquered by the socialist hordes of the eternal oppressors of the human race. Neither the abominable Hitler nor the bloodthirsty Stalin had even dreamed of going that far. Sometimes, I became very transcendent, but I always ended up laughing at it all. I didn't want them to think that I took it all very seriously. But still, they didn't know how to refute my arguments.

People in Glass Houses Shouldn't Throw Stones

I looked carefully for possible flaws that would dismantle the feeling of realism that the voices induced in me. Nothing nor anyone appeared to interrupt them while they rattled on mentally. It was as though each of them was isolated somewhere. Not all the characters were speaking all the time, but there were some very persistent voices, like *El Zumbao*. That was one of the reasons I guessed he was a lonesome beggar. The more aggressive they were, the more time they seemed to spend on me. Sometimes, I even noticed them being very angry.

I took my own behavior as a pattern. After all, I was also a telepath. I spent a lot of time quarreling with them. I was usually interrupted by some external event. I suppose that this happens to all of us when we're thinking about something for a long time. Did no one notice them being so angry? Did no one see them laugh for no apparent reason? Did their family and friends, as mine did, not ask them questions about their bizarre mood? They told me that their family and friends knew everything about the matter and agreed with them. I doubted it. Unless they were all as moronic as them.

I couldn't identify anything from myself in any of them. These people were not at all like any of the multifarious characters I usually made up. They had no personality traits that I found attractive. They seemed ordinary, even vulgar people and many could also be called nasty. Their methods were foolish: teasing, joking… their logic was simplistic, their morals were antics. How had they all come to my mind? Where did I get them from? I couldn't believe that they came from my brain, or from my environment. Nobody had tried to educate me that way; I didn't live in such a society either.

They seemed to take me for stupid. I couldn't deny that I did dumb things, some of them entirely boneheaded. I have never considered myself perfect and I always try to be self-critical. I'm prone to changing my personality traits when I don't like them, though often in an unwise way. But I was no more ludicrous than my voices. Their cocky attitude of superiority seemed a big mistake, and I often told them so. I tried again and again to get them to realize that they didn't have the necessary profile for me to consider them superior objectively. They were just arrogant, haughty, and ignorant bastards. Besides, I could call them this without feeling that I was insulting anyone whatsoever. It was a matter of fact. Anyone who observed the situation from outside would think the same as me.

Those telepaths talked a lot about respect; they demanded it; the respect cliché that everyone likes to claim and that I prefer to call consideration. Respect must be deserved; otherwise, it has no value. Respecting them, I would put my mother, for instance, on their same level. I used to tell them that their concept of respect resembled that of the Mafia. They saw themselves as the authorities, but they didn't think that they should also appear to be so. I told them that one respects those whom one admires and finds exemplary. For me, they were completely opposite to exemplarity. I compared them to the rubes in the fables, always ready to take their torches and pitchforks to slay the witch, the monster, or the weirdo. A vulgar lynching squad made up of a bunch of goons couldn't command respect from anyone. At best, they could cause fear. But, for that, they needed an essential requirement: a proof of existence. They had to prove they were real, that they could physically act against me. Not doing so was another big mistake.

To be honest, I felt that it was risky to be so insistent on this point. What if one day they decided to prove it to me? How would I take it if I knew they were all real people and could carry out their threats? When I wake up in the middle of the night, I usually look at the alarm clock to see what time it is. There are always some of them awake, too. Sometimes, it seems that it is I who wakes them up. In particular, *El Zumbao* is always awake. He never seems to sleep. Returning to when I look at the clock, I often think about what would happen if they told me the correct time before I could check it. Would it be a valid demonstration of their existence? Sometimes they do, and they usually give the wrong time, but it seems that they fail on purpose, as a joke. Occasionally, they have done something that could almost be considered as a demonstration.

When I watched the movie *Saving Private Ryan*, just a moment before getting to the scene where they finally find him, one voice told me: "Now, they find him." This left me puzzled, for I didn't know from where I could have got that information. Some trailer of the movie I forgot, maybe? It didn't seem like the most appropriate scene to use in a film trailer. They never did anything like that again. Sometimes, when I went to the cinema to a premiere, they'd say that I was a spoiler because they had not seen it yet.

They often tried to tantalize me, with a fatuous triumphalism that I found out of place, by repeating the tag-line I have chosen for the title of this book: "Thou shalt never get rid of us." I replied that they appeared to have more need to get rid of me than I had to get rid of them. It turned into a simple mutual annoyance, a childish fight. An eye for an eye and a tooth for a tooth. I was bothering them, and they would bother me. There was nothing to do, nothing to discuss or agree on. 'Death to intelligence!' it is said that someone said. The truth is that I also saw no way out. I had to learn how to live forever in this situation.

The Straw That Broke the Camel's Back

On our required weekend night outings, Bonita and I became regulars of one of the gay-friendly disco clubs in Chueca. We always ended the night there, staying until they closed, at 6 a.m. or even later. Some nights, we met folk who gave us good vibes and still wanted to party, so we continued the rave with them in an after-hours club.

Gays usually dress quite well. I really liked the way some guys dressed. I became a fashion victim, too; a metrosexual. I have always been tempted by fashion, but until then, I dressed in an inconspicuous, rather classic way, basically due to shyness. I wasn't very daring with colors. In this new environment, I felt liberated. I was on a steep learning curve as sometimes, my look was a real mess. It is not enough to buy two or three individual garments; one has to know how to combine them. It did not matter, because the milieu was of total freedom. Gradually, I was changing my gray wardrobe for colorful clothes, always adding something out of the ordinary. It was excellent therapy for overcoming taboos, shyness, and introversion. The night became the center and objective of my existence; I passed the working days waiting for the weekend to come, the actual life.

Since the voices were so moralistic and sanctimonious, when not being harsh and virile, I guessed that my new habits would inspire them to find other reasons for criticism and blame towards me. After all, I was moving within a sinful environment, Sodom and Gomorrah. "An atmosphere of fags," as I thought they would say. I have to say that they made some light attempts, but homophobia did not seem to be among their many defects.

It didn't offend me that they messed with my new friends. I know that a good part of society thinks that way, and, for me, they are no more than imbeciles. "It does not offend who wants, but who can," I used to tell them; "Don't tell me your opinions about people. It is none of my business," and other things like that. I had always worked hard to get them used to messing only with me. Other people had nothing to do with our particular personal war, and I was not going to allow them to involve my acquaintances. I used to tell them that, if I took into account the rabble's opinion about someone I liked, I would be bringing that person down to their level. As a result, it would be I who was offending, not them. For this reason, they did not take much trouble to criticize anyone other than me.

I was consuming only beer and energy drinks, although I was starting to drink more than I should. The voices did not like it, but, while I was partying, I was not in the mood for voices, so I ignored them. The rest of the week, they would try and compensate by criticizing everything I did at work or in my spare time. They became so exaggerated that they verged on the ridiculous. It didn't matter, they just wanted to bother me as much as they could.

In those days, the stores called Smart Shops came into vogue. They offered legal plant combinations that promised to be innocuous substitutes for the dangerous illegal drugs. I also became interested in the cultivation of other types of vegetables, in addition to marijuana. Specifically, I grew hallucinogenic mushrooms of the Psilocybe genus. I tried them once, and the experience was astounding, although a hallucinogen was neither a drug to use often nor to party. I stored them dried in a jar in the freezer, waiting for some other occasion; summer, perhaps.

Psilocybin didn't seem to affect the voices either. With the mushrooms, they continued as always, neither leaving nor changing their personality, their way of expressing themselves or thinking. It was only me that changed. I was perfectly aware that my body and mind were altered, but the voices weren't. They continued to appear not to be in my body. Sometimes they told me that the substances affected them. That was wherefore they wanted me to stop drinking and taking drugs, though I no longer believed them. It was clearly just chicanery.

Summer came, and the holidays with it. We returned to the same campsite in Sitges. We pitched the tent, reunited with friends and acquaintances from the previous year, and met new people. We were soon integrated into the small wonderful family that yearly formed there during the first fortnight of August. We went out partying that same night, and the next morning the voices also took their holidays, something that was going to become customary.

In the evenings in Sitges nights, like in so many places on the coast, the party atmosphere prevailed even more than in Madrid. In the clubs we frequented, there was not only dancing and fun but also sex and drugs, openly. I was tempted by the MDMA tablets, ecstasy, and Mi Niña became quite concerned given my past experiences with pills. I wasn't too worried about it, for I didn't attribute my delusions and hallucinations to sporadic consumption, but to excessive and continued intake. This began to create tension. For her, it was the never-ending story. She was getting fed up with the situation and didn't know what to do with me.

Summer passed, and we went back to our usual lifestyle in Madrid. We began to go out with one of Bonita's co-workers, a girl. This friend loved to smoke hashish and, moreover, she loved beer too. We were an explosive combination. I also started smoking hashish, apart from pot. Bonita was getting more and more sick of the situation. Sometimes, she would meet friends and ask me not to go with her, because she didn't want me to end up making a scene before them. We begin to drift apart. The situation came to a head on a Friday night. I had met our mutual friend for a drink. We were in a bar in the Lavapiés neighborhood, drinking and smoking joints, though not excessively. I can recall perfectly that I came back home by taxi. It left me in my doorway and I went up to my apartment, tipsy, but not drunk, went to bed, and fell asleep. The next day, Bonita was gone. She had not even left a note. I feared that something wrong had happened, but I had no idea what it could have been.

Time passed, and she neither returned nor called. I went out to buy some clothes and take a walk around the neighborhood to distract my mind. Lunchtime came, and I still didn't hear from her. I was becoming more and more concerned. By the evening, with no news yet, I went to sleep with a sinking heart. The next day, more of the same. I didn't want to leave the house in case she called on the phone. Eventually, she called and said she was coming back because we had to talk. She came back at night and told me the whole story.

She told me that I had woken up and gone to the bathroom. I must have been sleepwalking, for I didn't remember anything. Instead of going to the bathroom, I went to the fridge, opened the fruit drawer, and started pissing in there. Hearing the sound, she jumped out of bed and ran to pull me away, yelling at me and asking what I was doing. She said that I was spaced out, saying absurd things as if I was speaking in a dream. She put me in the shower, trying to wake me up. I had dilated pupils and just repeated over and over *"Dove l'acqua?"*. I think I must have been dreaming about an Italian friend we had met that summer in Sitges. There was no way to wake me up. She put me back in bed, and I fell asleep on the spot. The next day she woke up, took some clothes, and left without saying anything, just to think. I could not believe it. I thought she had dreamed it. I could recall coming home and going to bed, nothing more.

Mi Niña decided that she no longer wanted to live with me. She couldn't bear the situation any more. It had lasted a long time and was all too much for her. There was nothing I could do but agree with her. I didn't ask her to give me another opportunity. I didn't make the typical promises that I would change; I know myself too well. Nothing has ever hurt me as much as that moment and quite a bit of the time that followed. I collected everything in the apartment that could be used as a drug. I cut down the marijuana plants and threw them in the rubbish along with the dried weed, the hashish, the mushrooms, the ginseng… everything. I wept inconsolably for a long time, but she had already made her decision. We agreed that we would continue living together as friends until she found a place to go. Bonita couldn't afford the rent or take care of the cats, but I could. She only had a few things. She has never accumulated belongings, unlike me. I would stay in the flat with the cats. But living together was too painful. Finally, we decided that I would go to live with my parents for a month to give her time to look for something. I was lonely.

Journeys End in Lovers Meeting

The voices did not try to take advantage of my sadness, unlike what I was expecting. I don't remember them riling me about the matter. They kept bothering me, but they did it as usual. It was by then clear to them that they could only influence my thrills if I allowed it. I had several years of experience behind me. The key was not to develop any feelings of bonding with them, such as hatred or sympathy. I could protect my sadness from their intrusion and make it only mine. Moreover, that was when I started taking olanzapine.

Some friends told me that the phase of deep sadness would pass to give way to another one of resentment, which would end up in acceptance. I thought that the first of these phases would never end. She filled my mind, and I tried to see her as much as possible. I used any excuse to meet. For the first few days, I was obsessed, though at no time did I make any move to convince her to come back to me. I knew it would only spoil things more. It was better to settle for a possible future friendship though I felt unable to be a simple friend to her.

Neither she nor I stopped going partying. For me, that was an escape valve that I didn't want to give up. Since we kept going to the same places, we would meet each other. There were our friends and mutual acquaintances there so where else were we going to go? I quit drugs altogether, and my beer consumption dropped dramatically. I tried to drink as little as possible, perhaps three or four beers a night, and the nights were still long. After some time, the second phase, that of resentment, ended up kicking in. It seems that I am as normal as anyone else in this aspect. It was irrational bad blood; I knew I had no reason to be angry with her. In fact, it was the contrary. It was kind of my belief that the voices were real people: I know anger shouldn't have been there, but there was no way to get rid of it.

In any case, that helped me somehow to find relationships with other girls. One of those party nights, I ended up meeting another girl. She was much younger than me, and she was from outside Madrid. She studied at the university and shared a flat with a partner. Neither she nor I wanted to have any serious relationship, each of us for our own personal reasons, so I proposed a kind of open couple. We would see each other from time to time, and meet to go partying. The rest of the time, we would have a life of our own. Even so, it was something like a couple, and it was comforting. At the same time, it did not imply any serious commitment.

Bonita had rented a room at our mutual friend's home that she used as a help to pay the mortgage. In my heart, I kept hoping we would end up being together again, though I tried to resign myself to the contrary. The fact that she lived with our friend was an additional occasion for us to meet. After a while, we sometimes even went out together again as friends. We seemed destined to be together one way or another.

The relationship with my new 'girlfriend' had also got closer over time, although we were still a kind of open and independent couple. I kept trying to play fair with both of them: I didn't take any steps to get back with Bonita as I thought that this would end up taking her away from me. I told my new partner about all the flirtings I had with other girls, which, honestly, were not many. It began to seem not such a good idea to her. For my part, I also began to really feel attached to her.

Time went by. My life was divided between working and being away from home partying or having a drink on the weekend mornings. I used to go to El Rastro or another of the many bar areas in the center of Madrid. I went back to drinking more than I should. Although I tried not to go too far, spending most of the day going from bar to bar is enough to end up drinking too much. I had abandoned all my hobbies. I didn't read, I didn't DIY, I didn't play video games, I wasn't interested in television… I was only at home just enough time to take care of my cats – and they hardly needed care. I heated frozen food, cleaned, slept just enough, and little else. I lost hours of sleep so I could be out partying. Every Sunday morning I met with our friend and Bonita's landlady and her many acquaintances in the neighborhood, Lavapiés. I needed the company of people, but that lifestyle was exhausting.

I hardly found anything to talk about with many of these folks; we did not have any common interests. Sometimes, we'd meet each other and have a few beers, and, with the joy of the moment, we'd spend the rest of the morning together, to never see each other again. I used to mention the voices as a talking point. Strangers also didn't give a damn about the topic. No one ever asked me a question about it. It didn't seem to interest them either. Once, I got very angry with our mutual friend because she told me to stop trying to make people feel sorry for me by telling them that story of the voices. Apparently, I was the only person in this world who had a genuine interest in the phenomenon, a scientific curiosity.

People were only talking about mundane things. I was paying a high price in terms of health for all that vapidity. Luckily, this made me get back on course a bit. I stopped over-partying, which only provided meaningless relationships that led me nowhere. I stopped meeting that friend and began to see more and more of my new partner. Our relationship stopped being so open. And so it was about six months until the summer holidays arrived.

For me, the Sitges campsite was mandatory. Sometimes, I would joke with Mi Niña about this, asking her if, in summer, she would also follow me to Sitges. I told her it was a shame that she would miss it, and I was really sorry about that. We had both had a great time and had great friends there. They were the fifteen most special days of the year. But that year, she decided to change. Together with our mutual friend, she would go to another campsite in Andalusia, also on the beach. My new partner often said to me sadly, "You are still in love with her." I always said no, and I wanted to believe it. I needed it, for it had no sign of being fixed. And I wasn't going to try to force it.

I decided to go alone anyway, because there I would see my old friends again and meet new people, like always. At the last minute, my new girlfriend – for she had become almost that – came too. The first week she would come with me to Sitges. I arrived, set up the tent, and went to Barcelona to pick up my girlfriend at the Sants station. We had dinner and went out partying. The next morning I woke up without voices, as usual. I was already on holiday for real. Every day, we had a lot of parties. The environment was too tempting, so I started taking MDMA. It had no different effect than expected, with only a light hangover the next day. By day, beach, restaurants, and bars; at night, party and debauchery. And so, day after day.

The day before my girlfriend had to go back home, I received a surprise call from Bonita. The holidays with our mutual friend had not gone as well as she had hoped, and she wondered if I minded about her coming to spend the last week in Sitges. I told her: "Of course, you must." My girl said sadly: "You are going to get back together." I assured her we wouldn't. The next day, she left and She came. That night we went out partying. When we woke up, we were a couple again. We did not talk about it. There were no conditions. I think neither of us was quite sure, but there we walked through the campsite, holding hands again. All our friends were thrilled. We were the talk of the summer, worthy of the tabloids. Nor did she seem too concerned with my renewed fondness for ecstasy. The patient waiting had come to fruition. We never split up again.

Johnny, la Gente Está Muy Loca

When we went back to Madrid, we each went to our respective homes for the moment. I still couldn't believe it. I met with the girl who was now my new ex-girlfriend to explain the situation and break off the relationship. In the following days, Bonita and I spent more and more time together, until we decided that it was foolish to continue living apart. She gathered her things and returned to settle back in to her true home, with me. She brought with her a female kitten she had adopted, named Una Luna, who also joined the four of us. The voices, as usual, reappeared.

By then, the nightclub in Chueca where we used to go partying closed. At the same time, we started going out with two of Mi Niña's new colleagues and their many friends and acquaintances. They were all party boys and girls, very handsome and very fashionable. We changed disco pubs for discos: Ohm, Pasapoga, Cool, Polana… Sometimes, we even ended up in some after hours. When we went out, we took MDMA. In addition to MDMA, I sometimes took MDA, closely related to ecstasy, but which is taken orally in powder. We also took cocaine, although this was not my thing. I prefer to take a pill than have to go to the toilet all the time. That annoyed me and made me feel like a junkie. Neither of these drugs affected the voices, they only berated me a little more than usual, but they were not stoned.

One day, another strange character appeared, whom I also called *El Zumbao*. His entire talk was nothing but claptrap, although he used a pitch that made it clear that he was making fun of me. He wasn't laughing, but his voice sounded as if he was. He was persistent and annoying like a mosquito's buzz, the adult equivalent of a baby's cry. To the other, more rational voices, I could reply rationally to their teases, but this one didn't care about anything I said. "I love being a…!" he replied mockingly to whatever I called him. With him, there was no way to be sharp, unlike with the rest. I had no choice but to bear with the nuisance until he got tired. I had to acknowledge the effectiveness of his methods. I used to put him before the other voices as an example of a job well done. At least, so I could vex the rest. To bother me with no possibility of response, they should stop trying to use reason or intelligence. They were not prepared to use it.

The participation of the gang that I called *Los Garrulos* became more active. They used to suddenly address the others in a mocking voice: "The latest from Miguel…!" And they would explain, in their own way, what I was doing or thinking. They also had a different behavior regarding my vices. They used to encourage me to make mistakes instead of blaming me. Their goal seemed to drive me to do some crappy thing that would get me into trouble. The only chance against them was to attack their supposed manhood, break their protective testosterone shield. Sometimes I was pretty successful. I was becoming quite a makeshift psychologist.

In this way, another year passed. I became fond of electronic music: house, dance, techno, progressive… In parallel, I also got into doing some exercise. I am not interested in sports as a viewer, but I have always liked doing physical activity. I had long since neglected fitness, but my new metrosexual image required a body in line with it. I bought two dumb-bells and used them frequently.

Bonita got the idea of buying a flat. Becoming an owner did not appeal to me and nor did I want to leave the apartment we resided in, despite the tough times we had had there. Anyway, we looked for and found a flat. The new apartment was smaller, but it was ours. We made an additional renovation and moved to live there. All the computers were shelved in the attic corresponding to the flat. At that time, I had no other hobbies than music, bodybuilding, fashion, and partying. As the song says, I was one of those Loca people of the night.

Sixteen Tons

By focusing my life on holidays and weekends – the party – I ended up completely losing interest in my work. I needed it to afford that lifestyle, but I performed it reluctantly. Besides, I didn't have much to do. The working days seemed eternal to me, as though I were locked in a jail. I spent the day drowsy and bored shitless, counting the minutes until I could leave. I played Solitaire and Minesweeper on the computer, wandered around the Internet trying to find something entertaining, and downloading hundreds of songs. At that time, many platforms allowed almost anyone to be members of a huge band of pirates. But nothing interested me. I also lost interest in relating to my colleagues.

I fell into a kind of depressive state which was quite unusual for me as I always used to be active and interested in learning things. I would have lost interest even in the voices, had the telepaths not tried to exhaust my patience by endlessly reminding me they were there. The voices found fertile ground in my negative and irresponsible attitude towards work. My lowered mood seemed to give them wings as if they thought their time had come, for my defences were weak. Faced with this constant attack on my self-esteem and self-confidence, I focused on preventing the voices from fulfilling their objective, instead of correcting their reasons for criticism.

It should not be concluded that this confrontation was a piece of cake for me. It was a taxing and absorbing activity that distracted much of my mental resources. It wasn't easy to handle. They always had the recourse of saying that their objective was being accomplished anyway. They were stealing time from my life. They claimed they neither cared about anything

I said nor my opinion on what they said. My life didn't matter to them; my behavior was my business. They only criticized it to make me jumpy.

The only one who was making an effort was me. Neither I nor my health nor my beliefs mattered in the least. They detested me and wanted to make my life hell. They said I was a fool for listening to them. This, for me, was the worst-case scenario. It would leave me with no possible answer. If it was all a nihilistic attack, just because they disliked me, what could I do? Should I tell them that what they were doing was unfair? But the fact is that they were many and they devoted a lot of time and effort to me, too much for it to be a simple, pointless brawl. These reflections occupied my mind twenty-four hours a day. The first problem was the voices, the rest could wait.

This situation lasted for a long time without too many changes. The company was not at its best. The benefits were insufficient to offset the costs, and, little by little, we were going downhill. I almost wished it, though I was not clear about what I was going to do next. Some of my workmates left work, agreeing to a dismissal modality that would allow them to get the dole, but without compensation, since there was no money. The company could not even continue to pay wages. Other colleagues, in an attitude that was quite unfair to my bosses, insisted on staying on in their positions. They wanted the severance pay they were legally entitled to, so the company couldn't simply close. The atmosphere was increasingly rarefied. I also decided to leave, helping my bosses, who had helped me so much in the past. I was at home again, without a job, though with a good unemployment benefit that would last up to two years, in the worst case.

I spent eight long months diddling, reluctantly attending a few job interviews until I had to take seriously the need to work again. It didn't take long to find a job, and it wasn't exactly in a small company. It was a big company and they needed someone who had my knowledge and experience: I was proficient in the database management system they used and also their software development platform. This platform was already obsolete; therefore, it was difficult to find experienced developers. I got the job with ease. It was a promotion in terms of my future possibilities.

Take the Voices and Run

The long months of rest had a healing effect on my mood. The new office was also close to home and close to the Prado Museum. I had no need to get up early and could walk to work, through one of the most beautiful and stately areas of Madrid. A luxury. My stress levels went down, and the novelty and variety of the new job, in the industrial sector, made me gradually recover my liking and interest in my profession.

I had some remorse for having lost my reading habits, and I worked on getting them back. I couldn't read on the way to work, I only had nights for that, so I forced myself to look for a novel and try to overcome sleep for at least an hour every day. Another of the good habits that I acquired was to take physical exercise more seriously. The sedentary life I was leading was not the best for being fit and active. We joined a gym and started doing fitness regularly with our friends. I also bought some more weights and a mat so I could do some bodybuilding at home.

My weekend habits did not change, though. I had gone back to smoking tobacco, although I was considering quitting again. I bought a well-known self-help book that promised it was easy to quit smoking if you knew how to do it. It was a revealing book, for it helped me understand how anxiety works. I discovered that if one learns not to trigger anxiety, it is quite easy to quit smoking. Actually, this can be applied to any other drug, vice, or habit. I became interested in self-therapy.

Even so, on weekends, I continued partying and consuming alcohol and other drugs. Some voices still insisted that if I stopped doing so, they would disappear, and the problem would be solved. By that time, I doubted there was anything in this world that could end them. The medication only helped me to sleep, so I gradually decreased the dose down to the minimum.

This new situation lasted for about two years. One summer day, Mi Niña and I were in the pool. We heard two ladies talking about a relative who had gone to live far from Madrid and was very happy in his new destination. We had often played with the idea of going to live elsewhere, to Sitges, of course. Besides, the campsite we went to every year was about to close. Right there, we made the decision to move. The companies where we both worked had premises in Barcelona, and the two of us got the transfer. We would rent our apartment in the center of Madrid and, with the money, we would pay rent in Sitges.

At the end of another year of preparation, we found a fantastic apartment on the village's outskirts. Even the voices loved it: "It's a palace!" they exclaimed when we visited it. It was a flat overlooking a horse-riding field, with horses, geese, cats, and other animals, with the mountains in the background, almost in the middle of nature. On New Year's Day 2007, we moved excitedly to start a new stage, leaving behind the whirlwind of the big city. It was a great decision.

Réflexions Sur la Violence

We knew Sitges like the back of our hands since we had peregrinated to this beautiful Mediterranean town for ten years. We were friends of quite a few locals, and also had good friends in Barcelona. Adapting to living here was effortless for us; it was a dream come true. The campsite closed that same year. Clearly, we had no choice but to move to Sitges. The voices no longer disappeared, not even on holiday. A couple of years ago, that effect had ceased, perhaps because my enthusiasm for being there was no longer so intense. It didn't matter, because I had new incentives to become satisfied and confident. Things were going as planned, we were fulfilling our objectives and our life was improving.

The two of us worked in Barcelona, Mi Niña in the city center, and I in the industrial zone. That meant traveling on public transport for at least two hours a day. I got used to reading the free newspapers that were distributed in the morning at the station. I had to be in the office at 8 a.m., so I acquired the healthy habit of getting up early. I had a two-hour lunch, and thus, extra time to read. Soon, the newspaper became too small for me. I completely recovered the habit of reading and began to devour all my pending literature and new books that were appearing. This had a very stimulating intellectual effect. Reading became a necessity again. During the commuting, *Los Garrulos* used to accompany me, trying to annoy and vex me, in their ornery way, throughout the journey, to prevent me from concentrating. I used to counterstrike, trying to hurt their macho self-esteem. The fact is that they made me lose a lot of time, but many times I ended up managing to humiliate them and be the winner. The forces were yet balanced.

However, I felt that my effort, unlike theirs, was productive. I was investing time in reinforcing my personality. Although it is not very common to be involved in real life in such a situation, it is still important to be able to keep the composure in the face of pressure and psychological attacks from others. One has to learn to be assertive, but also to be something more if things begin to get rugged. We are a hierarchical species. Dominance is widespread among us, and many dominant people develop this trait in ways that tend to be abusive. It is a distortion similar to greed. It doesn't hurt to be capable of refusing attempts at abuse and getting bullies to walk away with their tails between their legs. They seemed to gain nothing more than the mere illusion of keeping a kind of old-fashioned honor, a stereotyped and clumsy virility. I, at least, could consider that I was going somewhere, growing as a person. They were on the worst side, that of the wrongdoers.

One of the realms in which I could not help but give them some reason was that of violence, physical violence. As much as one would be able to successfully maintain a verbal confrontation with another person, to impose oneself through arguments of any kind, there is always the resource of asking: "What if I give you a punch?" One can puff one's chest and start talking about barbarism and being above those things, but if the other strikes, the discussion is over and lost. Of course, I consider violence to be a weakness. The human being can compete, or even fight, with much more honorable and human traits such as ingenuity or intelligence, though the fact is that many people trust violence for the simple fact that it works. Violence is typical of monkeys, savages, or barbarians. It can only be successful in the short term, and it always ends up bringing adverse consequences. Mind you, don't tell that to someone who functions that way.

The voices didn't usually threaten to assault me physically. Nevertheless, sometimes I managed to rile and offend one of them enough to do it. I used to challenge them to come to Sitges, hoping I could see their faces at once. I laughed at them, saying that they would have to spend the whole trip arguing with me to keep their testosterone level high, though I kept thinking about the fact that I had no defense against a real physical assault. I could be strong enough, but I didn't know how to fight.

I have no doubt that the level of anger required to be able to fight would appear half an hour after the attack. I didn't expect a real attack from anyone, but I realized that this was a weak point. If you know how to defend yourself, regardless of whether you succeed, you can choose whether to do it or not and with what intensity. If you don't know how to defend yourself, you have no choice, and usually, you don't even react. I considered having some self-defence training. The goal was, above all, to cover that rift in my self-confidence. To not fight, one has to know how to fight.

My neighbor owned a gym. I paid him a visit, and he recommended I start with body combat. Body combat is like a kind of aerobics, but using movements from different martial arts. It is a very intense exercise; one learns to kick and punch, but only in the air, not hitting anything. It didn't take me long to be very fond of it. The key was to enhance everything that could be an intellectual or emotional reinforcement. I was still at war with the telepaths. A war that I couldn't afford to lose.

Though *Los Garrulos* used to predominate in the commute, the peeves were more varied at home. *El Zumbao*, any of them, used to lead the ruckus. Zumbao-one, with his usual tags: "Something must be done!", "He must have a weak point!", "You are going to have your comeuppance!", and his endless tirades about my behavior and my ideas. Zumbao-two, with his foolish nonsense. The rest of the troop, somewhat more rationally, used to interfere with my thoughts continually. "Don't you have a home? Don't you have family, friends? Isn't there anything on TV?" I asked them. It was almost routine, mere formalities.

In the miserable behavior of the voices, I recognized some traditional beliefs, customs, and dogmas. I often thought about it very critically. Criticizing cultural principles was much more productive than personal attacks; at least, it bothered them much more. If one wants to attack conventional people, it is best to attack their conventions, which often form a central part of their personality, of their identity. Our society has and has always had a lot of reasons for being criticized. We end up using even our best beliefs and customs for despicable purposes. I sneered at them that these issues seemed to interest me much more than them: 'Ye, its ardent and ill-prepared advocates.'

Sitges Mon Amour

Sitges is a very crowded place, especially at weekends. Just about at any time of the year, there is some event: the carnival, the International Fantasy Film Festival, the Barcelona-Sitges Rally of vintage cars, numerous fairs, and exhibitions. Also, it is a prominent tourist destination, a village visited by people from all the surrounding towns, and an iconic place for the gay community. Despite all of that, it is much less congested than the center of Madrid or Barcelona. To spend all year next to the Mediterranean sea produces a pleasant and continual feeling of being on holiday. It cannot be denied either that it is a beautiful and original town.

All of this induced in me a state of well-being that, in some moments, could almost be described as ecstatic. I was filled with satisfaction, elated. I savored every moment when I strolled through the alleys or the promenade, when I sat on a terrace for a drink, or when I partied at night on weekends.

When I was a child, I lived for several years in Barcelona and Figueras, in the province of Gerona. Visiting the surrounding areas always brought me fond memories of my childhood. Going to the beach to sunbathe as soon as the weather allows it, be it winter or summer, is a major luxury obtained almost at zero cost. If it is cold to lie on the sand, one can sit on the stairs that go down to the beach from the beautiful seafront to have a beer and watch the sea. The climate is milder than that of Madrid. The air is cleaner and healthier. I had the feeling of having ended up in paradise. "I have left the neighborhood," I sometimes thought to annoy Gasparín, in his already very few appearances.

At work, things were also almost perfect. The office was in a warehouse in Barcelona's Zona Franca, a place that is not pretty, but that is quiet. I had to take the train and a bus every day to get there, but they were not as crowded as in Madrid. I could almost always sit reading. My bosses were in Madrid, and my situation was one where I could go back to work as a freelance again. All my coworkers were very nice people, and we used to talk about many topics.

The work environment was also much more relaxed than that of Madrid. It is not that less work is done, but people are not as stressed as in the big capital, and that is transmitted in the atmosphere. My tasks were more varied than in my previous jobs. I also had to attend to the rest of the workers' computer issues, so I was in constant contact with people. This somehow compensated for my natural tendency to be inward looking. I'm not as shy as I was when I was a teenager, although I am an introvert.

Mi Niña was also happy in our new place of residence. The change of scenery even had the effect of improving her breathing. She has always had asthma, and here she was finally able to stop using inhalers every day. We both started taking fewer and fewer medications. Little by little, we stopped taking aspirin, ibuprofen, stomach protectors, allergy pills, cold tablets… I was still trying to stop taking – without success – olanzapine. I stopped going to the psychiatrist, and the olanzapine tablets were prescribed by the GP. I saw no point in going to a specialist, moving to another municipality, to tell them something that actually they didn't seem to care about. I stopped using ecstasy when I was partying at the weekends, but there were still some cocaine lines.

I used to drink no other alcohol than beer, though this didn't prevent the occasional inebriation. There were periods where I drank every day, interspersed with other times where I only drank at weekends. I stopped smoking – and restarted a few months later – lots of times. By then, it had been years ago that I had smoked my last joint. My friends in Barcelona were very fond of marijuana. The few times I fell to the temptation, I felt so bad that my desire died forever. We also started to like healthy and balanced food. It seems that reducing the level of stress remarkably and naturally favors the acquisition of healthy habits.

It might be thought that this whole bath of luxuriating and gratifying sensations should have had a noticeable effect regarding the voices, but it was not so at all. They didn't appear to be affected by that, either. They still seemed foreign to me. It didn't matter what I took or didn't take or how I felt. I wondered why they had disappeared every year during my short holiday, and whether there was a way to reproduce the situation. To what would it have been due?

Sometimes, they tried to keep me from sleeping. At night, the voices used to fade, as if we were all going to bed. It was like a sort of tacit agreement to allow everyone to rest. Some nights, I couldn't fall asleep, and I used to ruminate over some idea or I would mentally sing a song. Usually, the result was that I couldn't get things out of my mind and would just feel more and more awake. Then, the voices would get angry, saying that I wasn't letting them sleep, and swore revenge. Sometimes, in retaliation for some daytime brawl, they would attack me fiercely, make fun of me or talk about me enthusiastically to hook my mind and keep me awake. I'm used to answering them automatically, so many times I fell victim to their provocation. It can take me several hours to fall asleep then. I didn't use to give it much thought; things are how you take them. It was worse to provide them with useful resources. When I tried to quit the olanzapine, *El Zumbao* used to get angry, as if he wanted to force me to retake it. In fact, he urged me to retake it, insisting that I should not stop. That was not such a strange thing, because he always says I have to do the opposite of what I do.

Another annoying technique the voices use is to repeat everything that I think. Sometimes, one of them even says what I am about to say or think an instant before I am conscious of doing it. On other occasions, they speak at the same time as I do, or a little later. This always has a rather annoying outcome. It is like wearing headphones with which I hear myself speaking with some sort of delay. Actually, having access to the mind, it is not necessary to make any great intellectual effort to break one's balls.

If they also added an ironic or boastful tone, as if wanting to make their intentions very clear, the whole thing could become unbearable. However, they didn't do this often, though I never understood why. I suppose God shapes the back for the burden. I have read many stories of people who hear voices and have ended up overcoming the problem, and all of them are happy to have gone through the experience. I think now I am too, though back then I was not happy at all.

So two idyllic years passed, long enough for me to get used to the good life. It seemed that nothing could break the charm, that everything would continue like this forever, but it wasn't to be. It is not that anything too serious happened, only an important project for the company, and I was told that I had to return to Madrid indefinitely to undertake the development. I received the news like a hammer blow. I was going to be expelled from paradise and, besides, separated from Mi Niña for months. Anguish and rage came over me. How could I break free from this? The stress came back suddenly and multiplied.

Growing Up. A Mountain Out of a Molehill

It seems incredible how spineless one can become. Good life weakens the character. A fighter like me feeling impotent and overcome by a trifle. I even tried to get a medical certificate advising against the transfer, based on my mental disorder. But I couldn't avoid it, it was decided. I achieved an intermediate solution: I would go to Madrid on the AVE (high-speed train) from Monday to Friday and return to Sitges at the weekends. 'Things are how you take them', 'We suffer more often in imagination than in reality'. In Madrid, I could choose between a hotel next to the office or sleep at my parents' home. A luxury, free weekly trip to visit the family. I changed the absurd anguish for the determination to work in the most efficient way possible so that the situation would not last for long.

Going from feeling a kind of helpless victim to being determined and self-assured was a catalyst and a catharsis. I quickly got used to it once the project started and I moved to Madrid every week. I had to get up very early on Mondays to take the first AVE in the morning. I slept a little more on the train and went straight to the office. I worked tirelessly, with my mind focused so that everything was well designed and there were no bugs. I hardly talked to anyone; I just worked and worked. Later, I went to my parents' home or to the gym. The voices were over there, trying to annoy me, as usual, but I ignored them; I was not wasting time on bullshit. At weekends, there were great reunions with Bonita, for we both missed each other so much. I even started liking it.

Finally, I managed to get the job advanced enough to have prospects of being able to go on holiday and even return home permanently. Two train journeys a week required a significant reading supply. I had to buy some books to read in the many idle hours of travel. I wasn't looking for fiction, but self-help books and some easy and not too profound essays. By then, I only relied on self-therapy. One of the books caught my attention. It was about how to defend oneself against verbal attacks. I said ironically to the voices that now they were done for. They also didn't much trust what the manual could teach. I do not know if the explanations will be valid for the real world, I have never had to defend myself face to face from the verbal attacks of anybody, but it really wasn't useful to cope with the voices. Too naive.

Another book was helpful to me, though. It recommended using the great philosophers as a means of inspiration for self-help. It spoke about Socrates, Plato, Seneca, and the Stoics in general. Since high school, I had pending the project of delving into philosophy, but it seemed awkward and dense. This book encouraged me to lose my fear. There was another one that promised to tell the history of the world without the boring bits. It made me lose my fear of history, too, another of my pending topics. I always suspected it couldn't be as dull as it seemed. I apologise to the educational system, but there are so many unmotivated people who have a kind of allergy to fundamental and exciting topics such as mathematics, philosophy, or history, which is not what could be said to be a good sign. Ladies and gentlemen, school textbooks are dullsville, aren't they?

There were also some essays on current affairs that made less impression on me but made me get used to this type of reading which was more academic and thought-provoking. Some popular science works made me recover a taste and interest in science. I was cultivating the intellect anew. Although, for the moment, the weekends continued to be dedicated to the night. When you know all your friends will be out partying, when the only thing you do with them is going out, when meeting them during the day means doing the same thing you do at night, but with more light, withdrawing from the night is synonymous to withdrawing from the world. To this, we must add that this type of activity almost generates an addiction. As long as one has a great time, regardless of how damaging it may be, one wants to continue like this for all eternity.

The experience finally ended, just over three months after starting, in time for the summer holidays. It helped me to stop being so whiny and namby-pamby and, as a bonus, to begin a phase of personal growth. Some ancient peoples, such as Germans and Spartans, tried to avoid the vices of a good life. Philosophers like Diogenes, and philosophical schools like that of the Stoics, also made their attempts in this regard. They were all exaggerating, but they had a good eye.

There Are More Things in Heaven and Earth, Horatio...

I became a regular at the bookstores in search of philosophical readings. The first thing I did was to buy all Plato's dialogues and something from Karl Popper – I soon ended up acquiring almost all of his works. The considerable amount of references that these books contain allowed me to discover more and more authors and their major works. This type of reading became almost a vice, a healthy vice this time. I was very interested in epistemology, the philosophy of science, and through Popper, I got the most important works of many other prominent authors.

I spent most of my two-hour lunch breaks reading blogs on economics, law, and politics. I preferred to get my information from these than through the television news. They seemed much more serious and accurate. I also signed up for various philosophy forums on the Internet to maintain discussions with other people. In one of these forums, arguing with another member about logic, a third made a comment saying: "It is incredible how much a person can talk about logic when they have no idea on the subject." This was unpleasant, but he was right. So I began to study logic feverishly. I wasn't going to be an ignorant bigmouth in any realm. I ended up writing a couple of programs capable of checking the correctness of a logical argument. No one was ever going to call me ignorant rightfully any more. The continuous harassment of the voices gave me a kind of need to avoid being criticized for something that I could criticize myself for, too.

Given this, there are only two options: either you decide that you don't care about criticism, or you have to overcome your shortcomings. The former is easier than it sounds, 'Things are how you take them'. The latter is uplifting and nurtures personal growth. I learned to do both, as it suited me. Learning is a good thing from any point of view, the best investment one can do, so when lacking was ignorance, I always chose growth.

I was also fond of history. I discovered the Peloponnesian War by the hand of Thucydides, the founding of Rome and the Punic Wars from Titus Livius, the speeches of Demosthenes before the assembly, the Medical Wars and the exotic ancient peoples described by Herodotus, the conquest of Asia by Alexander the Great, the exciting Expedition of the Ten Thousand led by Xenophon, the decline of Ancient Greece, the fall of the Roman Empire in the exhaustive work of Edward Gibbon. I followed World War II, as written by Churchill, Eisenhower, Hitler, Rosenberg, and Goebbels themselves. I knew the horrors of the Holocaust, told by witnesses such as Víctor Klemperer or Rudolf Hoss, and the subsequent trial of the Nazi Eichmann analyzed by Hannah Arendt. I heard of Stalin's crimes, narrated by Solzhenitsyn; the First World War, the subsequent Versailles Treaty that led to the second, and Keynes' criticism and warning; our Spanish Civil War…

History led me to politics and economics. All subjects and all points of view were of worth to me. The more I was against something, the more I was interested in knowing everything about it, the more favorable opinions I sought, the more attacks and defenses I tried to find. My reading moments are a kind of dialogue – even a hectic discussion – with the authors and their ideas. I spend almost as much time reading as criticizing what I read. My mentality has been adjusting to the ideological conflict. I work hard to defend my position and to criticize that of the opposite.

I am immersed in a permanent rhetorical struggle with the voices, in a conflict that revolves around dominance and imposition. Culture is not just a beautiful thing, a kind of veneer of civilization. Culture can also be a weapon, a bloodless one that allows people to be free, for it prevents the mind from being captured and controlled by the interference of other minds. This, and not medication or drugs, became the right healing therapy. Knowledge has served for me as a defensive weapon and as a tool. I could never have written this book without it. I spent years playing with the idea before feeling able to do it. But it was time for the voices to start paying the rent. I'd make them earn the food I gave them!

Regarding my professional side, all this had a very positive effect. My knowledge was becoming obsolete again. I had to salvage it. My renewed and reinforced passion for reading, the kind of topics I chose, which were often hard, my taste for difficult challenges, led me to study maths. Data analysis is one of the booming fields today, and for this, mathematics is essential. Artificial intelligence became another pole of attraction. I started taking certification exams on different technologies. I made use of my free time to develop my own personal projects. Programming became a hobby again.

Since I am in the privileged position of being able to observe mental disorders from a personal point of view, psychology and psychiatry could not be missing from my now long list of favorite topics, and also the philosophy of the mind, a trending topic nowadays. I devoured popular science works on neuroscience: Damasio, Ramachandran, Pinker... Now I'm able to read academic papers at PLOS ONE. I have had to finally learn to master English to be able to read many of these works. By the way, this has given me an excuse not to abandon literature altogether, which I now read in English to practice and expand vocabulary. The fascination in these topics has led me to study biology and biochemistry too.

In for a penny, in for a pound. I have dabbled with physics – a subject that has always been hard for me – specifically, I'm very interested in chaos theory and complex systems. My home is full of books. I have to choose them carefully, for I have almost no room left on the shelves. Still, I can't help but buy more every month. I have got into the habit of getting up every day, without exception, at 6 a.m., sometimes even earlier, to dedicate as much time as possible to study and reading. I am self-employed again, working at home – a luxury. My room also looks like a mechanical workshop. My activities are back to being feverish, though this time without chemical help.

I have heard many times the saying 'Jack of all trades, master of none'. I don't think it's entirely true. A broad knowledge gives perspective on all things, and all things are related. There will always be something that interests you more or that you have to pay more attention to. Your job, without going any further. For me, the separation between science and letters is absurd. And it's not that I believe it, it's that I know it. Saying 'I am of science' or 'I am of letters' is equivalent to saying 'I am half ignorant'. Being ignorant is not an evil thing from an ethical point of view, it is only faulty in practical terms. It is also inevitable that the more one learns, the more one realizes it. In fact, becoming aware of how much you still have to learn, though paradoxical, is reliable proof that you are making progress.

The great figures, those we consider geniuses, have always been people with a broad culture and interests. Learning has also helped me to stop using drugs permanently. It didn't take much effort, it was enough to have something better to spend my time and mind on. The party and the drugs have definitely lost in the competition against personal growth and expansion. I sometimes still have one or two beers too many, but I like the result less and less. I have had to just fill life with something valuable that enables me to enjoy it fully. Relationships with others are also made easier and more fruitful. I have become more independent, and this allows me to socialize better.

Nowadays, there is a lot of emphasis on caring for the body. However, there is much less interest in caring for the mind. Everything in our body works because it is controlled by the brain. Exercising and following a healthy diet is essential, but if you don't help your mind to work, you are neglecting the most critical part of health. The main problem is always motivation. My great natural curiosity has been joined by the need to fight for control of my own mind. It is not easy, and, of course, it is wholly inadvisable to be involved in such a situation. Perhaps everyone should reflect on whether the fight for life provides them with the necessary challenges and incentives to motivate themselves to grow as a person. The famous comfort zone can become a death trap.

Sic Semper Tyrannis

My fondness for physical exercise grew even more. I spend many hours a week doing sports. I joined a gym where I could practice MMA, mixed martial arts. For the last two years, I have been practicing krav maga, a self-defense system. This has also helped to strengthen my personality and self-confidence. Knowing how to defend myself does not make me more aggressive but less. In short, I have become wiser and more complete, which has made me more and more at peace, albeit no less active. As time has gone by, I have more activities to carry out, more pending projects waiting to be done.

My thinking has become a continuous dissertation, a constant reflection on philosophical, political, and social issues. My profession is to solve problems. For this, I use logic. I have become very critical of everything done by the human being, and of the human being itself. All ideas, all beliefs are scrutinized and disassembled or improved by me. My way of thinking became very disruptive. I could mix ideas from all imaginable creeds while questioning each and every one of them in particular. They were all incomplete. They seemed more destined to separate than to unite, to manipulate than to liberate, to create manageable factions. I like to think of myself as an iconoclast.

For the voices, this was a constant source of trouble. They had always thought that, when I gave up drugs, I would become a normal person 'like them', and I would finally understand them and stop rejecting their claims. I always told them that neither were they normal people nor would my personality or my attitude towards them change at all, as it was. My intellectual development did not affect them either, in the sense that they remained without change; they seemed to learn nothing. They still appear to be people outside of me, determined to have some influence on my mind, to agree with me on the things I should or shouldn't do or think about.

There was no longer much to criticize in my behavior. The voices might have been satisfied. Even so, some of them kept on trying to impose on me their conventional and simplistic, politically-correct mentality. Their interference bothered me less and less; I began to tire of so much nonsense.

However, over time, there were changes in the behavior and attitude of the voices. *Los Garrulos* disappeared almost completely. Of the various *El Zumbao*, only one seems to be active still. He still spends time harping on with the rest of the voices about his "Something must be done!" or "He has to have a weak point!". Apparently, he is the only one left standing with claims that this absurd confrontation will continue. The other attackers appear from time to time, as in waves. I am not very clear about what these out-of-the-blue attacks are due to. They do not seem to follow recognizable patterns, as if they have been devised by other minds.

Some voices even agree with me quite often in my reflections. It has been a long time since they last said, "Thou shalt never get rid of us". Nope, apparently, but it also seems that this is not the only solution that can be given to the matter.

Unvollendete

Talking of conclusions on a matter that is not yet over might be somewhat premature. Science does not provide a satisfactory answer to explain the phenomenon of voice-hearing. In psychiatry, it is considered a symptom of psychosis or schizophrenia, just as pain is a symptom of infection. Talking about what the voices say is to fuel the patient's delusions, so only medication is used to try to eliminate them, with rather unsatisfactory results.

Luckily, in the 1980s arose the Hearing Voices Movement, with prominent figures such as Marius Romme, Sandra Escher, Mike Smith, and Ron Coleman, to name just a few, who consider unusual the phenomenon of hearing voices, but in principle normal. The disorder comes from the relationship established with the voices, not from the fact of hearing them. Psychiatry does not take into account the selection bias of meeting only patients who hear voices and have problems coping with them. People without trouble do not seek medical advice, and it seems that the proportion of people able to manage the matter by themselves is almost seventy per cent.

Anyway, we all move in the field of hypotheses. Nobody knows for sure what happens in our brain when we hear voices. Not all cases are alike, since there are different areas where activity may be correlated with the thing. Indeed, we don't even know yet how the mind is generated from neural activity. There can and should be many hypotheses, but we must be very clear that they are just that, to not perpetuate malpractice, as though we were abiding by unbreakable natural laws.

In this sense, medical dogmas themselves can also cause severe disorders. Sedating a patient almost to the point of being in a coma using tranquilizers is similar to the ancient practice of mixing an alcoholic beverage in the baby bottle to keep children quiet and calm. As with pain relievers, they are not a solution to a problem, just a relief, at best. I think that, fortunately, this situation is currently changing, though.

The approach focused on therapy and the exchange of information between people who hear voices – through international networks such as Intervoice – seems to work much better than the medication alone. In my first years as a voice-hearer, when I had the most significant problems with the phenomenon, I found little literature in Spanish on the subject, and there is still a lack of it nowadays. I found the website of one of these networks in Spain, albeit the activity was scarce, and soon it stopped working altogether. Recently, having improved enough my level of English, I have finally been able to read many of these books that I had pending, plus some others that have appeared over time.

The conclusions and hypotheses that I have read in all of them are very similar or identical to mine. The results obtained with this approach also seem much more promising for recovery rather than just medication, so I feel like this is the right way to go. Though virtual, it is a social problem; it is about interpersonal relationships.

I have talked to quite a few psychiatrists over the years. They have never tried to sedate me, for at no time have I shown them that I was not in control of the situation. I have always chatted with them as an equal. No one has treated me condescendingly, as if they were speaking to someone who does not know what is being said. They have never proposed sedative medication. The treatments they have prescribed have produced hardly any side effects, albeit they have not been effective either. It has never been suggested that I participate in any kind of therapy. Nor had any of them the slightest idea of how the phenomenon occurred.

I was often frustrated by their lack of interest in what I told them about the speech of the voices. I think they were not prepared to discuss the matter. I guess many are not even that curious about the subject. Probably, being intrigued is more likely in people who are devoted to research. I have always explained the phenomenon to doctors as I do it in this book. Rationally, I know, or rather I feel, that they can only be a product of my brain, but, at the same time, I'm not capable of eliminating the alternative beliefs. They didn't seem to have much to say to that. I guess as long as I claim they are hallucinations, everything is fine. I need to take olanzapine to sleep; otherwise, I would have stopped visiting a psychiatrist many years ago. I believe that some other people need more of their time than I do.

Living beings develop powerful mechanisms of adaptation to the environment. The conscious mind is one of these mechanisms, and it works continually adapting to a wide range of situations and circumstances. The voices also seem to have a high capacity to adapt to the environment. They can disappear due to changes in brain chemistry or intense emotional states, but they always end up adapting to the changes and returning. It seems that the only option is to adapt oneself, too. In that, everyone must find their way, although the help and support of others may be essential. But it is your mind, and you have to shape it and be the architect of the changes. Beliefs are the natural tool to achieve this, but, beware, they can lead to heaven or to hell.

The fact of thinking that they are telepaths, and at the same time, rationally considering that they cannot be that, seems inconsistent, but it is not at all. The mind is more than just pure reason. On the more basic emotional levels, I need a belief. The arguments that prevail are those capable of generating it. It is the belief that has the lowest energy cost, the one that best fits the need that demands it, the one that produces a more satisfying feeling. Our needs raise yearnings that we often try to calm through consumption or obsessive rituals. It is a natural mechanism, like that of hunger or thirst. One needs company, one needs to express oneself, one needs love… just as one often needs explanations.

Beliefs cover our need for explanations, especially in the absence of knowledge and the impossibility of obtaining it. They are somehow a kind of medicine and, as such, can also cause problems if abused; but if they are used responsibly, they fulfill their task without problems. That part of my mind that needs an explanation fits perfectly with the idea of telepathy. It is like keeping a child or animal happy with a harmless toy. I can consciously make all kinds of speculations about the physical impossibility of the phenomenon, about the absurdity of the situation. I can behave as if my voices were just that, hallucinations, objectless perception, but without the idea of the telepaths, I cannot deal appropriately with the issue. They seem to be people, so it's easier to act as if they were. Reason and logic only transport the truth, they do not create it. You cannot argue or fight with an entelechy.

The voices that assault the sense of hearing cannot be ignored all the time. This only creates stress, and stress feeds the problem.

This focus on beliefs has made me radically review my way of considering convictions, and that has had a very positive impact on the way I see the world and society. In the first stage, I have heard voices of known – and living – acquaintances. I believed that they were the ones who spoke, and I have verified that this was not the case. Later, they have been known neighbors. Then, others that were unknown have joined, and these were pure invention. Stranger, grotesque, and even ridiculous characters, but somehow they were credible to me. Finally, they have become telepaths, as the most natural explanation to accept. (What the heck is a hallucination? Think about that.)

Many people believe in gods that no one has ever seen. It has never been considered pathological – unless it was a god other than the official – and that has only been supported by general opinion. A simple myth about a miracle is enough to consider irrefutable evidence of the truth of those beliefs. Nobody sees the great religious infrastructures as the works of maniacs trapped in delirium. Nobody analyzes religious wars as aggressions among the alienated. Politics is also riddled with myths. Some of them have led to the greatest atrocities in history.

At best, only the principal leaders are labeled crazy, and only because we need an excuse to consider them different from us, their followers. The executing arms are often ordinary people. So, also, are the people who support, allow, and even collaborate to make those events happen. For a belief to be flagged as the result of delusion, a social convention, an authorized opinion, is sufficient. To be designated as the opposite, too.

Now, I see beliefs as mere mental tools. I produce them, and I can change them. Thus I am above them. I am responsible for them, but I am not at their service; instead, they serve me. I think the same about the beliefs of others; I am no longer convinced by anyone's opinions, I no longer feel compelled by any creed. My natural skepticism has triumphed, and it has done so based on beliefs about beliefs, metacognition. Knowledge is a challenging and laborious thing to acquire. Beliefs, conjectures, fill gaps that it is essential to fill. They are inevitable, but one has to be careful with them, feel responsible for them. As the tools they are, we must take care of them and keep them in good condition so that they are useful and harmless to us and to anybody else.

History has not been made only by good people, nor have good people always produced good works, and much less perfect ones. Many beliefs honest in origin have been used throughout history for perverse and manipulative purposes. Most contain even still today the imprint of these mistakes, of corruption, of abuse. The voices – mostly felt as alien to the listener –are, in essence, a social matter. They also use many beliefs in a tortuous way, trying to manipulate emotions and feelings. They rely on our natural social trait, on empathy, which makes it difficult for us to escape the influence of other people's opinions, what other people think of us. They use voice intonation to direct their emotions towards us.

The voice-hearer is the constant focus of attention of their particular chorus of voices. They are immersed in a community formed, sometimes, by oppressors, by aggressors. The struggle against the voices, at least in my case, is a social fight. I think it was wise to consider it a problem of socio-political and cultural relationships, for there are many ideological resources available to work in this area.

It has always been said – and I think with a marked ideological slant – that without firm beliefs that we can consider to be unquestionable truths, the individual is lost, and society will disintegrate. As far as I'm concerned, this is utterly false. Relativizing beliefs, not feeling bound by them as if they were transcendent principles imposed by higher instances, has made me feel more secure in myself, more in control. It has also made me feel more comfortable with others. I no longer see their beliefs as something dangerous to me, as something they could impose on me.

Training to refute the opinions of others, paradoxically, makes these opinions more acceptable. It even makes it a kind of sporting challenge. We are social by nature; we don't owe it to anyone. We need others for biological reasons, not just for practical purposes, and certainly not only to reinforce our beliefs, and much less our identity. My rejection of those I consider bad guys has increased, though, but I have raised the bar quite a bit in that regard. I have become utterly uncompromising when certain limits are crossed.

At the same time that I have achieved to understand other positions without sharing them, I have managed to learn to oppose those that I reject without violence. I am no longer a partisan. I consider that all ideologies are incomplete, that they defend too many spurious interests, that they are all made to separate and manipulate. I can objectively value all ideas, clean them from bad influences, and keep what is good about them. In general, it is not the ideas which are wrong, but the interpretation and use that we make of them and, above all, the actions that we believe they justify and the resulting consequences of committing them. I have become the owner of, the person responsible for, my opinions. I like when they match those of others, but I no longer need it. I believe that self-confidence is achieved in this way.

The fear of possible physical aggression has encouraged me to learn to defend myself also in this field. Now I can be a true pacifist, for I can choose whether to use violence. I no longer need to hide or seek shelter in the group; I own my identity. I need others as friends, colleagues, or co-workers. I am individualistic and social at the same time. I have only detached myself from ballast, barriers, and chains, from what prevents us from growing.

My approach is personal, and I do not intend to advise anyone, let alone anyone overwhelmed by their voices. My pride has always prevented me from either negotiating with or making any concession to my voices. My rebellious personality has made me consider submitting to any of their claims as unthinkable. I have always told them that doing something like this was something like death. Their attitude would never be rewarded, even if it was deposed. There is no negotiation with a gun on the table, and whoever put the gun there should never sit at the table again. Nor should his friends.

Behind every concession made to someone who has ever tried to use violence to achieve their goals lies its legitimation. If we allow violence to work, it will never stop being used. I know this is a kind of heroic, romantic insight, but it made me feel stronger against the voices. For me, it was a strategy that worked fine, but it can be a disaster for others. The voices counterstrike fiercely.

I have never met in person anyone who heard voices. Therefore, I have not talked to anyone about our shared experience. I have read online or in books all the recovery stories I know. The most common and successful approach is usually to 'accept the voices'. Instead of brawling with them, many people use a rapprochement strategy. They change the way they talk to their voices, their feelings and emotions towards them, and the voices often respond by doing the same. There is a hypothesis that voices represent – or are the consequence of – repressed emotions. They feed on our feelings, and we can manage them through thrills, while we learn to manage our own emotional states. The fight and the confrontation with the voices do not usually favor positive emotional states.

I once read something about this approach, but I never felt able to follow it, or perhaps I misunderstood it. Maybe this can only be done with outside help and support. My focusing has probably been very risky until I have succeeded. It does not seem sensible to recommend it, although it could be interesting as an object of analysis. In fact, I think that, in this matter, there are no universal recipes. Each person is a world, and each one's voices are part of that personal and particular world. One can be inspired by what others do, but you will always have to adapt your strategy to your own life experiences, to your personality.

There is only one strategy that I think can be successfully applied to all cases and to which we all end up turning: it is okay to seek external help, sometimes it is even essential, especially at the beginning, but improvement begins when one is able to take the whole thing over and lead one's own recovery. This is achieved by taking an interest in the phenomenon, studying it, and studying oneself, making it a vital project, training oneself to carry it out, and bring it to fruition.

The phenomenon of hearing voices is correlated with stressful situations. Many times, it is caused by severe trauma, such as sexual or physical abuse. Some people say that they already heard voices before these events occurred – most of them from childhood – as if they had already been born with voices. In these cases, the consequence of the trauma is usually that the voices become aggressive. Many times, the voice of the aggressor or aggressors is added to or replaces the existing voices. I have found almost no testimony like mine: voices induced by drug abuse, without any previous trauma. In my particular case, conditions of high stress and sleep deprivation were added to drug abuse. I have never been able to determine if they are the result of a brain injury or if drugs have awakened or trained a natural mechanism.

It seems that voices can be induced and also turned off. Perhaps neurons can form specific networks to build more than one personality, or partial personalities, in the same brain. It should not be forgotten that – leaving aside mystical ideas such as that of the soul – our own personality, the self, is an emergent property of neural activity. Our mind is generated by the cells of our body. It is optimal to centralize the control of our complex organisms. We also require very complex interaction with the environment. We can internalize the personalities of others to recognize them, and we can perform mental simulations of interactions with them.

The brain can possibly host several simultaneous minds, even if only the main one is in conscious control of the body. The mind seems to be a community of different mechanisms. It is more than the self. The self may be central, but it does not control everything. Communication with these 'pseudo-minds' could be established by sharing control of language centres with them. There is a rather rare condition called dissociative identity disorder, which consists of having several identities, different from one another, which take control alternately. It could be an extreme case of voice-hearing, in which all the personalities are capable of taking complete control in certain circumstances.

Other similar conditions are produced by brain injuries: the 'phantom limb' consists of continuing to receive sensations from arms or legs already amputated; the opposite effect is to feel one of our limbs as if it were someone else's.

Understanding all of this is not an easy task. By asking the wrong questions, one gets the wrong answers. Our mind has not evolved to understand and handle the kind of massive phenomena occurring at microscopic scales in the formation and functioning of our body. We have only been aware of its existence for a few years now. In cases of significant brain damage, our organism can get healthy cells to assume some of the functions that the dead ones used to do, and that can cause interferences. The network organization of neurons allows the construction of redundant pathways to perform various functions, ensuring robustness in the event of failures. We don't generate many new neurons in adulthood. However, the synapses are continually changing, making it possible to learn new concepts and skills, reinforce existing ones, or forget those that are no longer either needed or used.

Perhaps there is some biological mechanism that builds the connections that give rise to personality, and maybe this mechanism can be altered to generate parallel pseudo-personalities, something like branches. It could be a mechanism of repair or natural development of the personality – perhaps evolved to optimize the adaptation of the self to the changing environment. Voices could be the result of interference between this mechanism and that of 'learning the others'.

I have tried many times to get the voices to explain what they wanted. They appear very sure until I give them a chance to specify. Then, they seem lost as though not knowing what to say. It was clear that they wanted me to stop using drugs, but this did not seem to be their primary objective. Indeed, when I did stop for periods of time, they continued more or less with the same attitude. When I finally did it, their behavior improved, though many kept attacking or annoying. What they want seems to be something to do with my relationship with them, rather than with my habits. Maybe their attitude only depends on my expectations and on what I suppose they are going to do or say.

There are people to whom the voices give orders that they feel compelled to obey. In my case, there have been commands, but none specific. As soon as I asked them to be more precise, they refused to say anything. I challenged them to try to get me to obey one of their orders. I mockingly dared them to order me to do something dreadful. They never did. They were always ambiguous, even contradictory, in their claims or in their own explanation of what they were. As if I lacked the imagination to finish defining them.

Voice-hearing is a phenomenon that can provide interesting data on human psychology, the functioning of the brain, and the emergence of the personality, of the self, even of social relationships. Although the Hearing Voices Movement's approach seemed to be a significant advance over the classical psychiatry, I missed an interest beyond the therapeutic, a real field of scientific research on the origin of the phenomenon. However, as I was about to finish writing this book, I had the opportunity to read the book, *Can't You Hear Them?* by Simon McCarthy-Jones, which has made me change my mind. It seems that there are indeed numerous studies and investigations on the matter. Besides, real advances are being made in the knowledge of the issue. And it is not only pathological cases which are studied but also those of people who have never had problems coping with their voices. I hope I am not mistaken if, paraphrasing Werner Heisenberg, I can hopefully affirm that to understand what they are and where the voices come from, 'We only lack some technical details'.

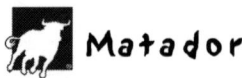

For exclusive discounts on Matador titles,
sign up to our occasional newsletter at
troubador.co.uk/bookshop